# To Improve Health and Health Care

## Volume VII

Stephen L. Isaacs and

James R. Knickman, Editors

*Foreword* by Risa Lavizzo-Mourey

# —⧈— To Improve Health and Health Care

## Volume VII

The Robert Wood Johnson Foundation Anthology

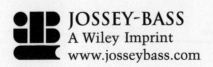

JOSSEY-BASS
A Wiley Imprint
www.josseybass.com

Published by Jossey-Bass
A Wiley Imprint
989 Market Street, San Francisco, CA 94103-1741    www.josseybass.com

Jossey-Bass books and products are available through most bookstores. To contact Jossey-Bass directly call our Customer Care Department within the U.S. at (800) 956-7739, outside the U.S. at (317) 572-3986 or fax (317) 572-4002.

Jossey-Bass also publishes its books in a variety of electronic formats. Some content that appears in print may not be available in electronic books.

ISSN available upon request.
ISBN: 0-7879-6823-4

Printed in the United States of America
FIRST EDITION
PB Printing   10 9 8 7 6 5 4 3 2 1

# –ᵚ–Table of Contents

     to Increasing Minorities in the Health Professions**    125
     *Jane Isaacs Lowe and Constance M. Pechura*

7    **The National Health Policy Forum**    147
     *Richard S. Frank*


## Section Three: Vulnerable Populations Portfolio    169

8    **The Injury Free Coalition for Kids**    171
     *Paul Brodeur*

9    **The Homeless Prenatal Program**    197
     *Digby Diehl*


## Section Four: Pioneering Portfolio    221

10   **The Robert Wood Johnson Foundation's
     Response to Emergencies: September 11th,
     Bioterrorism, and Natural Disasters**    223
     *Stephen L. Isaacs*

     **The Editors**    249

     **The Contributors**    251

     **Index**    259

# –ᴡᴡ–**Foreword**

Although The Robert Wood Johnson Foundation *Anthology* series contains many compelling chapters on the Foundation's initiatives to improve health and health care, perhaps its most valuable contribution is in demystifying the Foundation. It lets outsiders in on what happens behind the walls of our two-story office building in Princeton, New Jersey, as well as on the collaborative thinking in which we engage with our grantees. Since this is my first Foreword to the *Anthology*, I would like to help further demystify the Foundation by explaining our new priorities and how we arrived at them.

The Foundation has a rich tradition dating back to 1972—one that is evident from the approaches to grantmaking examined in this year's *Anthology*:

- Our approach of testing strategies that address important health problems is demonstrated by chapters on the Teaching Nursing Home Program (which aimed at improving chronic care by linking nursing homes and nursing schools), the Fighting Back program (which supported community coalitions to fight substance abuse), Join Together and the Community Anti-Drug Coalitions of America (two organizations that provide assistance to community anti–substance abuse coalitions), and our efforts to contain rising health care costs.

- Our approach of educating health professionals and those in a position to affect policy is shown by chapters on the Foundation's Clinical Scholars Program (a postresidency fellowship that offers physicians training in social sciences, public health, and health policy), the National Health Policy Forum for members and staffs of Congress and the executive branch of the federal government, and an array of programs designed to attract minorities to the health professions.

- Our approach of helping the most vulnerable segments of our society can be seen in chapters on the Foundation's injury prevention programs (which strive to reduce injuries to children living in poor inner-city neighborhoods) and the Homeless Prenatal Program (which provides information and services to homeless pregnant women and women recently released from jail).

- Our approach of looking for innovative ideas that can improve health and health care is evident from the Foundation's response to September 11th, and our response to public health emergencies more generally.

As the Foundation's new president and chief executive officer, I wanted to draw on the strengths of our traditional approaches while working with the staff and the board to hone them, and to develop new ways to meet the health and health care challenges of today and tomorrow. Shortly after I took office, I asked members of the staff to think about developing a limited number of specific, measurable objectives for the Foundation. After considering the matter and consulting with outside experts, staff members circulated their ideas and discussed them at an all-day meeting. I then met with the Foundation's senior staff to consider all the ideas on the table and to determine which to select. The priorities were presented to, and adopted by, the trustees in January 2003.

Out of this intensive analytical process came a modest but important refinement of the Foundation's goals and a new set of priorities. The new goals remained basically the same as the old, but with more emphasis on the importance of providing high-quality care. As modified, the current goals of the Foundation are

1. To assure that all Americans have access to quality health care at a reasonable cost

2. To improve the quality of care and support for people with chronic health conditions
3. To promote healthy communities and lifestyles
4. To reduce the personal, social, and economic harm caused by substance abuse—tobacco, alcohol, and illicit drugs

To meet these goals, we have developed an approach we call our "impact framework." It allocates our grantmaking across four "portfolios," much like those of a mutual fund complex that has different portfolios appealing to the varying objectives of individual investors.

- The first of these is our targeted portfolio, which is designed to address systemic problems in health and health care. Although recognizing that the problems we have chosen to address are complex and multifactorial, the Foundation will—through a combination of demonstrations, training, communications, and research—concentrate on discrete parts of problems with potentially measurable outcomes. This will allow us to better judge our impact. This portfolio includes nine focused objectives, four of which are designed to improve health (behavior and conditions that influence people's health status) and five of which are designed to improve health care (medical care and the system that undergirds it). Each of the targeted objectives has a defined time limit, running from two years in some cases to a decade in others. The targeted objectives that relate to improving health have to do with smoking, public health, obesity, and alcohol and illegal drugs. Those that relate to improving health care have to do with health insurance coverage, quality of care, racial and ethnic disparities, end of life care, and nursing.

- The second is our human capital portfolio. Through this portfolio, we plan to train leaders and to improve the health and health care workforce through programs such as the Clinical Scholars Program, the Health Policy Fellowships Program, and the Investigator Awards in Health Policy Research program.

- The third is our services for vulnerable populations portfolio. This portfolio continues and expands upon the Foundation's programs, such as Local Initiative Funding Partners, Faith in Action, and Cash and Counseling, that serve people in need. This portfolio takes a more direct approach by supporting programs that help people immediately and that develop and disseminate effective strategies that can serve those most vulnerable in our society.

- The fourth is the new pioneering portfolio. Through this portfolio, we will fund innovative, high-risk ideas and approaches that do not fall into any of the categories above.

To implement the new framework, we modified the Foundation's staffing structure slightly. Previously, the Foundation had been organized along the lines of program management teams—groups of between five and fifteen staff members from program, communications, research, financial, and legal offices—charged with developing and monitoring programs in a specific area. Since the team concept seemed to work for us, we decided to keep it, but to reduce the number of teams in the targeted portfolio from eleven to nine, each corresponding to one of the strategic objectives. The three remaining portfolios—human capital, vulnerable populations, and pioneering projects—are staffed similarly. Each has a program management team responsible for developing and monitoring programs.

Thus there is a lot of ferment within The Robert Wood Johnson Foundation: new leadership, new strategic directions, new staffing patterns. With so many changes coming at once, it is important to remember that we build on a very solid programmatic base, and that analysis of our past and current efforts, through the *Anthology* series and other means, can serve to guide our actions in the future. We are just at the beginning of a process that will, I expect, enhance the work of the Foundation and its grantees to improve the health and health care of all Americans.

*Princeton, New Jersey*                                   Risa Lavizzo-Mourey
*August 2003*                                              President and CEO
                                        The Robert Wood Johnson Foundation

# –⟪–Editors' Introduction: Observations on Grantmaking from The Robert Wood Johnson Foundation *Anthology* Series

Unlike business, where the goal is to make money, the job of foundations is to give away money. While businesses try to earn a financial return on investment, the return on a foundation's investment is measured by contributions to the public good. The basic tools of business are products (which can be ideas or services); the basic tools of foundations are grants and the communication of information accumulated by their grantees. Investing for financial return is not the same as investing for social return. Thus, while business can offer models and ideas for foundations—particularly in matters of managerial efficiency—the most useful ideas and models come from foundations themselves and the work of their grantees.

With this in mind, we have scoured the seven volumes of The Robert Wood Johnson Foundation *Anthology* series to find out what its seventy-five chapters reveal about the craft of grantmaking: What distinguishes effective from ineffective grantmaking? What approaches have led to a strong social return on the Foundation's investments? and why? The following are our observations.

## –⟪– Catching the Wave

The Foundation has enjoyed singular successes by entering fields about to emerge and helping to guide their development. Back in the 1970s—a time when, because of their size, hearses doubled as ambulances—an underground of medical professionals began to appreciate the need for a better emergency medical system. The Foundation stepped in and, working with the federal government, played a critical role in providing direction for the new emergency medical response system.[1] In the early 1990s, as the toxic effect of cigarettes was attracting the attention of health professionals and the media, the Foundation entered the tobacco field and helped shape one of the nation's more successful public health movements.[2] Similarly, through its early recognition of the potential importance of nurse practitioners and physician assistants, the Foundation helped that field take off and guided its development.[3] The same can be said of the Foundation's end-of-life programs, which in the 1990s helped harness a movement that had been gathering steam since the 1980s.[4]

One can never know, of course, which fields will take off and which won't. But the best program officers and foundation leaders will have a sense—through their conversations, reading, and travels—about emerging trends. (Sometimes, in fact, The Robert Wood Johnson Foundation's interest in an emerging field can give it attention that it otherwise might not have had.) Currently, for example, there is a lot of buzz around obesity, public health, and aging—three priority areas for the Foundation. If the past serves as prelude, the Foundation might be able to catch the wave and help guide the development of these areas.

## —ᗡ— Keeping Strategic Focus

In a large sense, The Robert Wood Johnson Foundation is focused. It awards grants only in the areas of health and health care, and it does not fund basic research or international projects. Its mission guides the Foundation's grantmaking.[5]

Taking this sense of clear direction down a notch or two—to priority areas and to programs—has been a challenge. Even with a relatively limited focus on health and health care, there is a dizzying array of ideas from which to choose, and it is easy to jump from issue to issue.

Where the Foundation has been clear in establishing the directions it wants to go (that is, where it has set clear objectives and goals) and then stayed with them, it has increased its chances of having an impact. Take two areas where the Foundation has had an important influence. In the case of tobacco, the Foundation honed in on kids' tobacco use early on, giving its grantmaking a clear focus. In its end-of-life programs, the Foundation concentrated on palliative care—again giving it a relatively sharp focus. In contrast, where the approach has been less targeted—where the Foundation adopted a more scattershot approach—the results have not always been as solid. The strategies for improving the care of chronically ill people, for example, have not been cohesive, nor have the results of the Foundation's efforts been as impressive.

As Risa Lavizzo-Mourey writes in the Foreword, the Foundation is trying to come up with a limited number of measurable strategic objectives for each of its priority areas. If these prove effective, they will give the Foundation (and the public) a clearer idea of where the Foundation is going and whether it is achieving what it set out to.[6]

## —⁗— Maintaining Tactical Flexibility

While it is certainly true that focus matters—that clear objectives and well-wrought implementation strategies are essential elements of success—it is equally, or even more, important to maintain flexibility in the tactics employed to attain long-term strategic goals.

Nowhere is the need for flexibility more evident than in the programs, mounted in the 1990s, to improve access to care. The Reach Out program, for example, which encouraged physicians to volunteer to serve the uninsured, emerged just as managed care was forcing physicians to work longer hours and cut back the time they had to volunteer. Many Reach Out sites responded by coming up with innovative strategies that allowed doctors to serve uninsured patients.[7] Similarly, the Strengthening Hospital Nursing program, designed to give nurses more clout in hospitals, was rolled out as managed care was forcing hospitals to cut their nursing staffs. Some of the program's sites showed great ingenuity in finding ways to circumvent this difficult situation.[8]

Nor are these the only examples. The National Program Office of Coming Home, a program set up to make loans to nonprofit development companies to build affordable assisted-living housing, discovered that borrowers needed money for up-front start-up costs, not the long-term permanent financing that had been originally planned. With the Foundation's approval, the National Program Office quickly changed the nature of the loans.[9] Similarly, when Join Together became the National Program Office for Fighting Back, which supported community anti–substance abuse coalitions, it revamped a plan that had looked good on paper but was not working in practice.[10]

## —ᴡᴡ— Staying the Course

In general, the Foundation has had a good record of staying with programs over a period of years, particularly in areas that reflect its basic values. For example, in the 1970s, it funded programs designed to increase the attractiveness of generalist medicine, and it maintained its support in the 1980s and early 1990s, even though the concept remained unpopular within mainstream medical practice.[11] Its work to advance minorities in the health professions has continued since the early 1970s,[12] as have its Clinical Scholars and Health Policy Fellowships programs[13] and its efforts to expand health insurance coverage.[14] The Foundation's commitment to these areas over a long period of time has given it an influence it might otherwise not have had.

The Foundation does, however, terminate its support for programs and, indeed, to entire fields of endeavor. After all, it doesn't make sense to stick with unworkable concepts—or to fund successful programs—forever. As former Foundation president and chief executive officer Steven Schroeder noted, "You've got to know when to hold 'em and when to fold 'em."[15] In many cases, the timing of decisions to end support appeared to be appropriate—mental health, cost containment, and some areas of chronic care come to mind. In other cases, the exit was probably premature. There is a widespread feeling that the Foundation's support of nursing and dentistry in the 1970s and 1980s ended early and that staying the course would have increased the Foundation's effectiveness.[16] The Foundation began supporting both fields again in the late 1990s and early 2000s.

While the Foundation has not found the secret of how long to stay (nor has anybody, for that matter), it has learned that a few years is probably too short a time to have a meaningful impact. As Foundation president and chief executive officer Risa Lavizzo-Mourey notes in the Foreword, the Foundation has now established time periods for each of its strategic objectives.[17]

## —w— Embracing Fields

The Foundation tends to take on big problems—like improving access to medical care, reducing substance abuse, getting people to exercise. One way it does so is by building the field.

When the Foundation does get involved in field building, it seems to be particularly effective when it embraces (in the sense of a bear hug) the problem by using all the tools at its disposal. Take, for example, the Foundation's work on smoking. It funded research, public policy dialogues, communications, demonstration projects, training, standard setting, advocacy groups, the Center for Tobacco-Free Kids, and the like.[18] A similar bear hug approach appears to have worked in the case of end-of-life care. As Ethan Bronner noted in his chapter in volume VI of the *Anthology*, the efforts of The Robert Wood Johnson Foundation and the Soros Foundation to legitimize palliative care demonstrated the power of foundations to nurture new fields.[19]

The approach, however, hasn't worked yet to reduce the number of people without health insurance coverage—an issue of great concern to the Foundation. The difference may lie in the nature of the problems. Take tobacco, for example. Smoking is widely recognized as harmful; there is a villain (Big Tobacco), and there is a simple solution (stop—or don't start—smoking). In contrast, the uninsured are not yet a matter of national concern; great differences of opinion exist on potential solutions to the problem; and health insurance is highly charged politically.

## —w— Supporting Talented People

The payoff from supporting good people and promising leaders is a recurring theme throughout the pages of the *Anthology* series. The Foundation supports people in basically three ways.

One way is by developing the capacity of those in the health field—as in its fellowship programs such as Clinical Scholars, Health Policy Fellowships, Scholars in Health Policy Research, and the Minority Medical Education Program[20]—or, as in the case of the Community Health Leadership Program,[21] by recognizing and supporting the work of leaders at the local level. Within The Robert Wood Johnson Foundation, there is a widely shared feeling that these programs to develop human capital have been productive investments, even though it's hard to prove.[22]

Another way in which the Foundation supports talented people is by giving them a series of grants over a number of years, thus allowing their work to mature and develop. David Olds is a good example. The Foundation first supported his work to train nurses to provide home visits to low-income pregnant women back in 1978; more than twenty years later, the Foundation continues to support Olds's work.[23] Olds is just one of a number of people whom the Foundation has supported year after year. The list includes Barbara Barlow, a physician at New York's Harlem Hospital, whose work to prevent childhood injuries the Foundation has been funding since 1988,[24] and Judith Miller Jones, the first and only director of the Washington, D.C.–based National Health Policy Forum, which the Foundation has supported since 1973.[25]

A third way the Foundation looks to support talented people is by awarding them (or, literally, their organizations) a grant based on a sense that they will get the job done. Former St. Louis Cardinals catcher Joe Garagiola, for example, almost single-handedly carried a program to reduce the use of chewing tobacco by enlisting major league baseball in the campaign.[26] Martha Ryan, a San Francisco nurse practitioner, received an almost unheard-of two grants from The Robert Wood Johnson Foundation's Local Initiative Funding Partners program to work with homeless pregnant women and with women newly released from prison.[27] Rhonda Roland Shearer, a New York City sculptor, received quick Foundation support for her efforts to bring supplies to rescue workers after September 11.[28]

At a time when carefully crafted objectives and measurable goals are given priority in the world of philanthropy, it is well to remember, too, that the Foundation's support of good people doing good things has reaped great dividends.

## —៱៱— Thinking Small—Sometimes

The Foundation has long taken pride in—and to an extent earned its reputation through—its strategic grantmaking in large demonstration programs. Some demonstrations have been replicated widely;[29] others have been models for government programs or legislation;[30] and still others have catalyzed or guided the development of emerging fields.[31]

But even though large strategic demonstration programs can be dazzling in scope and effect, the Foundation's programs that affect people directly form an important and often unappreciated part of its portfolio. Recovery High, for example, was an innovative New Mexico high school for substance-abusing high school students.[32] The awards made under the Faith in Action program support community volunteers who ferry elderly people to doctor's appointments and seniors' activities.[33] The Foundation's Local Initiative Funding Partners program actively seeks small community-based projects.[34] As one example, the Homeless Prenatal Program, which received funding under the Local Initiative program, provides needed services to women who often fall outside of the health care system.[35]

These programs and projects are not designed to change health or the health care system. They do, however, touch individuals directly, and this is important. Moreover, they win friends for the Foundation and keep its staff in touch with the reality of people's lives. Effective grantmaking balances the strategic with the charitable.

## —ɯ— Exploiting Failure

Everybody loves success and to build on success. Indeed, The Robert Wood Johnson Foundation sometimes tries to replicate successful programs and to "take them to scale" nationally. However, it's also important to admit and learn from failure.

The *Anthology* series examines a number of programs that have failed and areas that have not taken hold in the consistent and coherent fashion they were expected to. In some cases, the Foundation simply accepted the outcomes and moved on to other things.[36]

In other cases, it learned from failure and found better approaches to the problem or issue. Perhaps the best example is the development of the Foundation's end-of-life programs. Between 1989 and 1994, The Robert Wood Johnson Foundation funded a study, whose acronym was SUPPORT, designed to improve the care of terminally ill hospitalized patients by improving communications between physicians, nurses, patients, and patients' families. At the time, it was the costliest program the Foundation had ever funded. SUPPORT was a failure. Care of the dying patients did not improve, even after specially trained nurses had made intensive efforts to see that patients' wishes were honored.[37] Rather than hiding the failure or being discouraged by it, the Foundation took the opposite tack. Recognizing that the original problem still existed, it mounted a major and more diversified effort to improve care toward the end of life.[38]

## —⟋⟍— Recognizing Messiness

The Foundation has made investments in communities and state and local governments that haven't panned out, largely because the Foundation has not appreciated the difficulty and the messiness of bringing about change at the local level.

Foundation-supported programs that attempted to weave disparate, often competing, elements into community coalitions have not, as a general rule, met their objectives. Two examples are the Fighting Back program and the Community Programs for Affordable Health Care initiative. The authors of *Anthology* chapters examining these programs agree that one of the main reasons that they did not work was the Foundation's failure to appreciate the very real and practical difficulty of getting often-competing groups to work together for the common good.[39]

Similarly the Foundation's efforts to improve health policymaking at state levels foundered because of the Foundation's trying to impose order on a basically disorderly system. As Beth Stevens and Lawrence Brown observed in their chapter on the Foundation's efforts to improve health policy at the state level, "Foundations and those who evaluate their work should recognize that discussion, better staffing, technical aid, and diffusion of knowledge can tidy up the messiness of health politics only so far."[40]

## —⟋⟍— Utilizing Research and Communications

The Robert Wood Johnson Foundation devotes a substantial amount of its resources—both human and financial—to research and communications and to integrating them with program development.[41] Within the Foundation, there is an implicit belief in the power of research to provide knowledge that will lead to better policies and programs and the power of communications to put information in the hands of those who will use or benefit from it.

The investments in research and communications over many years have, in fact, given the Foundation—directly and through its grantees— a credibility, influence, and access that it might not otherwise have had. These investments have also provided a great deal of public information on many aspects of improving health and health care—everything from medical malpractice to workers' compensation and from tobacco policy to health insurance.[42]

Despite the value of the Foundation's use of research and communications, the *Anthology* series is replete with examples where research findings were ignored, where programs were developed without waiting for research or evaluation results, and where policymakers had the best information available but did not use it.[43] In a system that is not wholly rational, even the best research and the most strategic communications efforts may produce limited results.

Perhaps the lesson is that the Foundation's large investments in research and communications have paid dividends by giving the Foundation credibility and access, by providing the public (including policymakers) with timely and reliable information, and by developing a network of highly skilled researchers and communications experts. However, to the extent that research and its dissemination are ignored or overtaken by events (which, not surprisingly, happens frequently in the politically charged arena of health and health care), the return on investment is diminished.

## —〜— Taking Programs to Scale

An ideal for The Robert Wood Johnson Foundation is the small, well-evaluated, and widely publicized demonstration that is replicated at many sites and is ultimately adopted nationally. The ideal was reached in the cases of emergency medical services, nurse practitioners, training of dentists to serve disabled patients, regional perinatal networks, and, to an extent, palliative care and injury prevention programs.[44] More often, the ideal is not reached—hardly surprising, since large-scale social change does not come easily. What accounts for the difference? Why can some programs be taken to scale and others not?

One explanation of the difference has to do, simply, with timing. It is not coincidental that many of the successes occurred in the 1970s, a time when the federal government looked for programs to adapt and expand nationally. In the first years of the new century, the federal government has devolved responsibility for social programs to financially strapped states, which, in turn, are trying to pass responsibility to localities. The model is not as likely to work today as it did yesterday. Insofar as it can be made to work, it requires catching the wave, bringing all the Foundation's resources to bear, and engaging other foundations and, to the extent possible, governments.

Another reason for the difference has to do with the clarity and appropriateness of the model to be replicated. In the case of nurse practitioners, for example, despite variations in training and deployment, the model was relatively simple and repeatable. The same was true of regionalized perinatal care. In the case of AIDS, however, the community-based model based on the successful San Francisco experience turned out to be inappropriate for other locations that didn't have San Francisco's unique population and resources.[45] In the case of David Olds's nurse home visitation program, the original model using public health nurses to visit pregnant women in their homes was expensive, and the use of less-qualified personnel turned out to be less effective.[46] Whether the pure or diluted model should be replicated wasn't clear. Thus, clarity, flexibility, and appreciation of local circumstances are important factors in taking seemingly successful models to scale.

Finally, there is the matter of collaboration. Since only the federal government has sufficient financial resources to fund programs on a large scale, collaboration among foundations is needed for programs to be widely replicated. Yet foundations have shown little ability to work together in the past and have few incentives to do so in the present.[47] Taking programs to scale might require a change in the inner-directed culture of foundations.

—ɯ—

Foundations play a unique role in American life. Yet little is known about how to develop effective grantmaking strategies. Business, as we noted earlier, offers an imperfect model; because their goals are different, what works in a corporate boardroom may be wrong for a foundation headquarters. While there is no single right way to practice the craft of philanthropy, we believe that much can be learned from the successes and failures of a foundation with more than thirty years' experience.

| | |
|---|---|
| *San Francisco* | Stephen L. Isaacs |
| *Princeton, New Jersey* | James R. Knickman |
| *August 2003* | Editors |

## Works Cited

All citations are from this volume or previous volumes of *To Improve Health and Health Care: The Robert Wood Johnson Foundation Anthology.* Previous volumes are cited in the Notes as *"Anthology,"* followed by the year of publication.

Isaacs, S. L., and Knickman, J. R. (eds.). *To Improve Health and Health Care 1997: The Robert Wood Johnson Foundation Anthology.* San Francisco: Jossey-Bass, 1997.

Isaacs, S. L., and Knickman, J. R. (eds.). *To Improve Health and Health Care 1998–1999: The Robert Wood Johnson Foundation Anthology.* San Francisco: Jossey-Bass, 1998.

Isaacs, S. L., and Knickman, J. R. (eds.). *To Improve Health and Health Care 2000: The Robert Wood Johnson Foundation Anthology.* San Francisco: Jossey-Bass, 2000.

Isaacs, S. L., and Knickman, J. R. (eds.). *To Improve Health and Health Care 2001: The Robert Wood Johnson Foundation Anthology.* San Francisco: Jossey-Bass, 2001.

Isaacs, S. L., and Knickman, J. R. (eds.). *To Improve Health and Health Care, Vol. V: The Robert Wood Johnson Foundation Anthology.* San Francisco: Jossey-Bass, 2002.

Isaacs, S. L., and Knickman, J. R. (eds.). *To Improve Health and Health Care, Vol. VI: The Robert Wood Johnson Foundation Anthology.* San Francisco: Jossey-Bass, 2003.

## Notes

1. Diehl, D. "The Emergency Medical Services Program." In *Anthology* (2000).
2. Hughes, R. G. "Adopting the Substance Abuse Goal: A Story of Philanthropic Decision Making." In *Anthology* (1998).
3. Keenan, T. "Support of Nurse Practitioners and Physician Assistants." In *Anthology* (1998).
4. Bronner, E. "The Foundation's End-of-Life Programs: Changing the American Way of Death." In *Anthology* (2003).
5. Schroeder, S. A. Foreword to *Anthology* (1998).
6. Foreword to this volume.
7. Wielawski, I. M. "Reach Out: Physicians' Initiative to Expand Care to Underserved Americans." In *Anthology* (1997).
8. Rundall, T. G., Starkweather, D. B., and Norrish, B. "The Strengthening Hospital Nursing Program." In *Anthology* (1998).
9. Alper, J. "Coming Home: Affordable Assisted Living for the Rural Elderly." In *Anthology* (2000).
10. Chapter One in this volume.
11. Sandy, L. G., and Reynolds, R. "Influencing Academic Health Centers: The Robert Wood Johnson Foundation Experience." In *Anthology* (1998).
12. Chapter Six in this volume.
13. Chapter Five in this volume; Frank, R. S. "The Health Policy Fellowships Program." In *Anthology* (2002).
14. Holloway, M. Y. "Expanding Health Insurance for Children." In *Anthology* (2000).
15. Schapiro, R. "A Conversation with Steven A. Schroeder." In *Anthology* (2003).
16. Keenan, "Support of Nurse Practitioners . . ." (1998); Brodeur, P. "Improving Dental Care." In *Anthology* (2001).
17. Foreword to this volume.
18. Kaufman, N. J., and Feiden, K. L. "Linking Biomedical and

Behavioral Research for Tobacco Use Prevention: Sundance and Beyond." In *Anthology* (2000); Orleans, C. T., and Alper, J. "Helping Addicted Smokers Quit: The Foundation's Tobacco-Cessation Programs." In *Anthology* (2003); Diehl, D. "The Center for Tobacco-Free Kids and the Tobacco-Settlement Negotiations." In *Anthology* (2003).

19. Bronner, "The Foundation's End-of-Life Programs" (2003).
20. Colby, D. C. "Building Health Policy Research Capacity in the Social Sciences." In *Anthology* (2003); Frank, "The Health Policy . . ." (2002); Chapters Five and Six in this volume.
21. Mantell, P. "The Robert Wood Johnson Community Health Leadership Program." In *Anthology* (2003).
22. Isaacs, S. L., Sandy, L. G., and Schroeder, S. A. "Improving the Health Care Workforce: Perspectives from Twenty-Four Years' Experience." In *Anthology* (1997).
23. Alper, J. "The Nurse Home Visitation Program." In *Anthology* (2002).
24. Chapter Eight in this volume.
25. Chapter Seven in this volume.
26. Koppett, L. "The National Spit Tobacco Education Program." In *Anthology* (1998).
27. Chapter Nine in this volume.
28. Chapter Ten in this volume.
29. Chapter One in this volume; Keenan, "Support of Nurse Practitioners . . ." (1998); Brodeur, "Improving Dental Care" (2001); Holloway, M. Y. "The Regionalized Perinatal Care Program." In *Anthology* (2001).
30. Bronner, E. "The Foundation and AIDS: Behind the Curve but Leading the Way." In *Anthology* (2002); Brodeur, "Improving Dental Care" (2001); Rog, D. J., and Gutman, M. "The Homeless Families Program: A Summary of Key Findings." In *Anthology* (1997).
31. Diehl, "The Emergency Medical . . ." (2000); Keenan, "Support of Nurse Practitioners . . ." (1998); Lynn, J. "Unexpected Returns: Insights from SUPPORT." In *Anthology* (1997) (end-of-life care).
32. Diehl, D. "Recovery High School." In *Anthology* (2002).
33. Jellinek, P., Appel, T. G., and Keenan, T. "Faith in Action." In *Anthology* (1998).

34. Wielawski, I. M. "The Local Initiative Funding Partners Program." In *Anthology* (2000).

35. Chapter Nine in this volume.

36. Colby, "Building Health Policy . . ." (2003); Dentzer, S. "Service Credit Banking." In *Anthology* (2002); Rundall, Starkweather, and Norrish, "The Strengthening . . ." (1998).

37. Lynn, "Unexpected Returns . . ." (1997).

38. Bronner, "The Foundation's End-of-Life Programs" (2003).

39. Chapter One in this volume; Chapter Three in this volume (see the section on Community Programs for Affordable Health Care).

40. Stevens, B. A., and Brown, L. D. "Expertise Meets Politics: Efforts to Work with States." In *Anthology* (1997).

41. Knickman, J. R. "Research as a Foundation Strategy." In *Anthology* (2000); Karel, F. "'Getting the Word Out': A Foundation Memoir and Personal Journey." In *Anthology* (2001).

42. Newbergh, C. "The Health Tracking Initiative." In *Anthology* (2003); Berk, M. L., and Schur, C. L. "A Review of the National Access-to-Care Surveys." In *Anthology* (1997); Kaplan, M. S., and Goldberg, M. A. "The Media and Change in Health Systems." In *Anthology* (1997); Cantor, J. C., Berenson, R. A., Howard, J. S., and Wadlington, W. "Addressing the Problem of Medical Malpractice." In *Anthology* (1997); Dembe, A. E., and Himmelstein, J. S. "The Workers' Compensation Health Initiative: At the Convergence of Work and Health." In *Anthology* (2001); Gutman, M. A., Altman, D. G., and Rabin, R. L. "Tobacco Policy Research." In *Anthology* (1998); Weisfeld, V. D. "The Foundation's Radio and Television Grants, 1987–1997." In *Anthology* (1998); Garland, S. B. "The Covering Kids Communications Campaign." In *Anthology* (2003).

43. Diehl, "The Emergency Medical . . ." (2000); Chapter One in this volume; Knickman, "Research . . ." (2000); Alper, "The Nurse Home Visitation Program" (2002).

44. Diehl, "The Emergency Medical . . ." (2000); Keenan, "Support of Nurse Practitioners . . ." (1998); Brodeur, "Improving Dental Care" (2001); Holloway, "The Regionalized . . ." (2001); Bronner, "The Foundation's End-of-Life Programs" (2003); Chapter Eight in this volume.

45. Bronner, "The Foundation and AIDS . . ." (2002).
46. Alper, "The Nurse Home Visitation Program" (2002).
47. Isaacs, S. L., and Rodgers, J. H. "Partnership Among National Foundations: Between Rhetoric and Reality." In *Anthology* (2001).

# –ɯ–Acknowledgments

The Robert Wood Johnson Foundation *Anthology* is the result of the efforts of a great many talented individuals, whose contributions we would like to recognize.

We express our gratitude to those staff members of The Robert Wood Johnson Foundation who contributed to the book in a variety of ways: to David Morse for his invaluable insights, helpful suggestions, and sound guidance; to Risa Lavizzo-Mourey for her ideas on topics and structure, her support of the *Anthology,* and her comments on the manuscript; to Molly McKaughan for her astute editing of the chapters; to Deb Malloy, Sherry DeMarchi, and Nancy Giordano for their superb administrative support; to Paul Moran and Tim Crowley for their efficient handling of contractual and overall financial matters; to Carol Owle, Ellen Coyote, and Mary Castria for ensuring that specific accounting matters run smoothly; to Richard Toth and Julie Painter for their care in checking facts and figures (Julie is leaving the Foundation, and we will miss her careful reading of the manuscript); to Hope Woodhead for the professional way in which she oversees the book's distribution; to Barbara Sherwood for managing the distribution of reprints and making sure that copies of the book are available in the Foundation's lobby; to Hinda Feige Greenberg, Kathryn Flatley, and Mary Beth Kren for their research help; and to Linda Bilheimer, Victor Capoccia, Carol Chang, Steven Downs, Susan Hassmiller, and James Ingram for having reviewed various chapters.

Outside of the Foundation, we owe a great debt to the external review committee—Susan Dentzer, Frank Karel, William Morrill, Patricia Patrizi, and Jonathan Showstack—for their thoughtful reading of the manuscripts and sound comments; to C. P. Crow, whose editing improves every chapter; to Lauren McIntyre for her conscientious efforts entering data; to Carolyn Shea for her fact-checking; to Ruby Hearn, Paul Jellinek, Mathy Mezey, Martha Ryan, Steven Schroeder, Peter Shaughnessy, and Pauline Seitz for their comments on drafts of chapters.

At Health Policy Associates, Inc., we wish to thank Greta McKinney for her financial oversight. Finally, we would like to express our special appreciation to Elizabeth Dawson for her care, conscientiousness, and professionalism throughout the eighteen-month process of going from a series of ideas to a published book.

S.L.I. and J.R.K.

# To Improve Health and Health Care

## Volume VII

# Targeted Portfolio

# 1

# The Fighting Back Program

*Irene M. Wielawski*

## Editors' Introduction

In the mid-1980s, the use of illegal drugs among young Americans had created a social crisis in the nation. Crack cocaine was being sold openly in many urban neighborhoods, and the nation was attacking the problem largely through a punishment and interdiction strategy. But this was not working, and there was a general sense of despair that nothing would make a difference. In response to the crisis and to restore a sense of optimism, in 1989, The Robert Wood Johnson Foundation launched a program called "Fighting Back" to fight substance abuse by reducing the demand for drugs and, as it evolved, treating substance abusers. Through the 1990s, the Foundation authorized a total of $88 million for this program, which ended in mid-2003.

Fighting Back focused on establishing community coalitions composed of a broad range of local citizens, agencies, and organizations that would work together in combating the problem of substance abuse. The concept emerged from the 1960s War on Poverty and became popular among philanthropies in the 1980s as a way of encouraging bottom-up solutions to social problems. The

Robert Wood Johnson Foundation continues to fund a range of national programs that are built around the concept of coalitions.

One of the most ambitious national programs ever initiated by the Foundation, Fighting Back was complex, messy, long-lived, and controversial. It engendered passion from the program officers who created it, the grantees who made it happen, and the evaluators who studied it. An evaluation released in early 2003 reignited a smoldering controversy about the program and more profound underlying issues, such as whether a public health approach to fighting substance abuse is appropriate, whether community coalitions are an effective intervention, and how to evaluate community substance abuse programs. Even now, there is little agreement about what the program set out to accomplish and whether it succeeded or not.

This chapter by Irene Wielawski, a veteran investigative reporter who formerly worked with the *Los Angeles Times,* recounts the story of Fighting Back in all its richness and controversy. It provides an excellent case study of the tension and difficulties in mounting, implementing, and evaluating complex local initiatives.

T wo events catapulted thirteen-year-old James into the ominous embrace of a street gang: his parents' divorce and the loss of a cherished berth on the junior high football team in Vallejo, California. It was the beginning of his descent into drug dealing and mayhem. "I wanted to belong," he explains. "You know, to be one of the guys."

Now a high school senior and antidrug activist, James (not his real name) marvels at how matter-of-factly he arrived at such a bad decision: "I was pretty immature, I guess." He was not uninformed, however. Even at thirteen, James knew it was a risky path. He'd gotten all the right messages at home, school, and church. His family is part of the tight-knit Filipino American community of Vallejo, which, according to James, puts tremendous pressure on kids to excel. Gangs and those they attract were exactly what he was raised to shun. So James had some qualms and briefly thought of confiding in an older sister. But the emotional seesaw ruling his life in that bitterly unhappy period landed the other way. Concluding that his sister would "just lecture me," James chose the gang. To prove his merit, he began selling marijuana to classmates. The descent began.

Fortunately, it didn't go far, thanks to Youth Partnership, a community group in Vallejo that is part of a national substance abuse intervention called "Fighting Back: Community Initiatives to Reduce Demand for Illegal Drugs and Alcohol." Launched in 1989 by The Robert Wood Johnson Foundation, Fighting Back hoped to test the theory that by targeting prospective *users* with prevention and treatment programs, instead of simply sending police after dealers, the seemingly insoluble problem of substance abuse might finally be subdued. Vallejo, a blue-collar city about thirty miles northeast of San Francisco, was one of fourteen test sites in eleven states.

James had no idea he was part of an experiment. He went to Youth Partnership meetings simply to please his sister, who was a team leader. Unexpectedly, through peer discussions about taking charge of one's life, he found there the stability and sense of belonging he'd longed for. "A lot of my advisers talked about integrity," James recalls. "Basically what that came down to was you can't do what you are telling other people not to do."

James took this to heart. First he stopped selling marijuana. Then he started steering other kids who he thought were headed for trouble to Youth Partnership. Then, under Youth Partnership's auspices, he began writing articles for the local newspaper about the illegal drug and under-age drinking scene in Vallejo. "I never thought anyone read them, but kids did, and they said they agreed with me," James says. "Then my friends told me that I was their role model, and that made me feel good."

Looking back, James considers himself lucky to have found these community programs. "Youth Partnership and the Fighting Back Program really changed the direction I was going in," he says. "Basically, they changed my life."

———ɯɯ———

You can't get better testimony than that for a substance abuse intervention. But it begs several questions for those charged with finding effective community-based strategies against drug and alcohol abuse, such as the following:

- Can James's turnaround be legitimately credited to Fighting Back, when he himself lists his sister and upbringing as influential factors?
- How do you prove it?
- What if you can't?

Such issues of causality and proof undergird a debate about Fighting Back that continues vociferously even as the fourteen-year, $88 million experiment comes to a close. The Fighting Back program set out to test a number of theories, among them whether community coalitions are an effective way of combating substance abuse. And, in the way the experiment played out, questions remain about whether such programs can be considered successful if they help some people, such as James, but don't result in a population-wide reduction in substance abuse.

At the national level, Fighting Back's architects remain at odds with those responsible for evaluating it, who concluded that the program had no measurable impact on population use of alcohol and illegal drugs. Fighting Back proponents argue variously that the evaluative methodology was flawed, that it was fatally underfunded, and that it measured the wrong things. Meanwhile, at the local level, among Fighting Back's fourteen test communities, there remain widely divergent views about substance abuse interventions generally and the Fighting Back program specifically. These views are strongly held; exasperation verging on anger colors the debate at every level.

"Why all the heat?" mused Steven Schroeder a few weeks before his retirement in December 2002 as president and chief executive officer of The Robert Wood Johnson Foundation. Fighting Back wasn't his idea, but Schroeder presided over most of its tempests. If Fighting Back did not make an overall dent in substance abuse, does this by itself condemn the concept of arraying community coalitions against the problem—a fundamental tenet of the program? Many of those who participated in the coalitions would answer, resoundingly, "No!" As Schroeder bore witness, Fighting Back's evaluation is only the latest in a long series of controversies that have beset the program since its inception in 1989.

To what degree are Fighting Back's results rooted in the Foundation's program design? How much can be laid at the feet of what hindsight clearly reveals to have been an unrealistic implementation strategy? How much had to do with problems of leadership so severe that, at the national level, the Foundation had to replace both the first evaluator and the first program director, and only two of the fourteen sites stayed the course with their original directors. A growing pile of papers and analyses testifies to the search for answers to these questions. But here's another one: Is the untidy end of Fighting Back simply a reflection of the messy social context of alcohol and illegal drug abuse?

## —⚭— Why Even Go There? The Robert Wood Johnson Foundation Takes on Substance Abuse

Crack cocaine was new to most Americans in the 1980s, when the media began to chronicle its ravages on the front pages of newspapers, on the six o'clock news, and in graphically descriptive magazine cover stories. Crime and violence, damaged babies, degraded lives. For those who had reared children in the 1960s and 1970s, when marijuana and psychedelic drugs loomed as the greatest threat, the emergence of crack cocaine seemed ominous indeed. The result was widespread alarm over harm to the nation's youth and a general perception that "the drug problem" was out of control.

Enter The Robert Wood Johnson Foundation or, rather, the board of trustees of The Robert Wood Johnson Foundation, which surprised management and staff with a call for action on drug abuse. Typically, ideas for new initiatives in philanthropy come from staff members, many of whom are hired because of scholarship or experience in fields targeted by a particular foundation. But in 1986, when the trustees first voiced concern over the drug problem, The Robert Wood Johnson Foundation's primary focus was traditional health and medicine. It had neither staff nor programmatic expertise in substance abuse. This was the "Just Say No" era, to use the slogan popularized by former first lady Nancy Reagan. Embedded in the slogan were two messages reflecting the political mood of the country: use of addictive substances is a matter of choice; and if you choose to break laws concerning illegal drugs or irresponsible alcohol use (driving while intoxicated, for example), punitive consequences will result. Most substance abuse initiatives back then originated with the federal government, and about 70 percent supported law enforcement, as opposed to prevention and treatment.[1]

Ruby Hearn, a former senior vice president of the Foundation, and Paul Jellinek, a former vice president, drew the assignment handed down by the trustees. Hearn remembers being at a meeting at Meharry Medical College in Nashville when she got a call from her boss at the Foundation. The trustees, she said, had requested an antidrug initiative; Hearn's assignment was to head the in-house drug abuse task force. Separately, a task force on alcohol abuse was established. Hearn recalls scrambling to come up to speed on the drug field and, in the process, discovering "great confusion among programs and research initiatives at the federal level."

"Some of these agencies didn't even talk to one another," according to Hearn. "We learned that some of the using population had multiple problems, but if they had a drug problem, they had to go to one agency; if they had an alcohol problem, they had to go to another agency; and if they had a related health problem, they had to go to yet another agency. People said if you could possibly bring all of this activity under one roof, it would be a big help."

Jellinek, who worked with Hearn on the design of Fighting Back, found equally fragmented efforts at the local level. "What struck me was the incredible cloud of despair that hung over all the efforts from the White House down to the community level," he said. "No one knew what anyone else was doing, and nothing seemed to be working."

Bringing things under one roof quickly became a core tenet of Fighting Back, codified in the program's 1989 call for proposals. The Foundation envisioned a unity of purpose in the substance abuse field that had never existed. Essentially, it called for a truce among factions that had been not only separate but competitive and, in some cases, antagonistic. The Foundation expected advocates of twelve-step recovery programs (the Alcoholics Anonymous model) to mend fences with proponents of inpatient chemical detoxification. Community and business leaders were expected to find common ground with police, mental health, and public health officials. Residents of drug-infested, crime-ridden neighborhoods were challenged to commence a dialogue with the addicts they blamed for their troubles.

Fighting Back's architects believed that by getting all these people to work in concert, the demand for alcohol and drugs could be reduced population-wide. In other words, the *disorder* of the substance abuse field combined with the public's contentious and fragmented view of alcohol and drug abuse might be to blame for previous interventions' poor results. Fighting Back's design reflected classic public health thinking, albeit with an economist's twist—the notion that reduction in demand would discourage suppliers more effectively than police action.

The Foundation boldly declared these challenges to the status quo, then promised to put its results to the most rigorous scientific analysis. According to the call for proposals, communities that participated in the experiment would be expected to show a measurable reduction in substance abuse that could be credited to the Foundation's innovative strategy: coordinated community action to reduce the market for alcohol and illegal drugs.

The Foundation laid out its strategy and made clear that communities would have no leeway in how they organized their community coalitions. This rigid mandate from Princeton to fourteen disparate sites with unique social, political, and ethnic infrastructures disappeared in a subsequent reorganization of Fighting Back, at which time decisions on governance were left to the participating communities. But in 1990, the Foundation believed this was the only way to solidify the "under one roof" approach. "To ensure that effective coordination does occur," the call for proposals read, "the applicant will be required to establish" the following:

- "A citizens' task force on drug and alcohol abuse to provide oversight, guidance, and support. The task force should represent all groups in the community whose involvement and commitment will be needed for the initiative to succeed: parents, clergy, tenant groups, business and community leaders, health professionals, school superintendents, principals, judges, chiefs of police, elected officials, and others."

- "A community-wide consortium of all of the institutions, organizations, and public and private agencies whose participation is required to implement the proposed initiative, including the news media, civic and religious organizations, schools, businesses, major health care providers, human service agencies, drug and alcohol treatment providers, and others. Applicants should bear in mind that close coordination with local government and law enforcement authorities is essential. Also, the direct involvement of the relevant state agencies, as well as private insurers, will be key to addressing both immediate and long-range project financing."

How to hold these entities together was left to the communities' wisdom, as was the specific means to address substance abuse. In these areas, the Foundation gave Fighting Back communities broad latitude, acknowledging the diversity of substance abuse threats. Although Foundation action on substance abuse had been sparked by the crack cocaine epidemic, crack use wasn't pervasive in the United States. In some communities, heroin was the dominant threat. In others, it was methamphetamine. There was also variation in the populations seen to be at risk for substance abuse, whether youth or homeless people or a specific ethnic group. For example, one Fighting Back site, Gallup, New Mexico, chose to make alcohol its primary target, because of the historic toll alcohol abuse had taken on the region's Native American population.[2] So even though the Foundation mandated a single, all-inclusive approach for the structure of community coalitions, it gave the Fighting Back communities considerable leeway in setting priorities and in the specific approaches to achieving the goal of substance abuse reduction.

The carrot was potentially $3.2 million in funding to each of the sites selected: $100,000 annually for up to two years of planning, followed by $3 million to achieve the desired results. In response to the call for proposals, 331 communities applied to participate in Fighting Back. Of these, the Foundation, in 1990, awarded planning grants to Charlotte, North Carolina; Columbia, South Carolina; Kansas City, Missouri; Little Rock, Arkansas; Milwaukee, Wisconsin; New Haven, Connecticut; Newark, New Jersey; Northwest New Mexico (Gallup); Oakland, California; San Antonio, Texas; San Jose, California; Santa Barbara, California; Vallejo, California; Washington, D.C.; and Worcester, Massachusetts. Two years later, all but San Jose received implementation grants of $3 million each.

These communities set out to field-test the Foundation's assumptions: that broad-based community collaboration was possible on an issue lacking societal consensus; that ordinary citizens would accept a public health definition of substance abuse; that alcohol and illegal drugs are comparable ills; and that clandestine behavior can be credibly measured. In 1996, after a major restructuring of the program, funding for six projects was discontinued, while the eight remaining each got another infusion of $3 million. This second round of funding ended in December 2002 with Fighting Back's official close. But, according to the National Program Office, anti-drug-and-alcohol programs initiated under Fighting Back continue in New Haven, Charlotte, Kansas City, Milwaukee, Gallup, San Antonio, Santa Barbara, and Vallejo.

## —w— Fighting Words over Fighting Back

In early 2003, Leonard Saxe of Brandeis University completed his evaluation of Fighting Back. Using household telephone surveys, Saxe's team found no statistically significant decrease in illegal drug and alcohol use in Fighting Back sites as compared with demographically similar communities. The data, according to Saxe, hold up within individual sites as well as program-wide. The findings challenge the notion that citizens' groups can effectively decrease the use of drugs and alcohol across a community—the guiding principle of Fighting Back and one that has been widely adopted by federal and other agencies in similar initiatives. "There is no pattern of differences that lead you to the conclusion that these community-based coalitions are either a necessary or sufficient condition to reduce alcohol and drug abuse," Saxe says.

These are fighting words to Fighting Back's foot soldiers, many of whom insist that their communities have been changed for the better. They point to an array of accomplishments, including improved public dialogue and understanding of substance abuse, coordination of previously disjointed services, and new ventures aimed at dissuading alcohol and drug use or at helping addicts kick their habits. And some grantees flatly reject Saxe's results, expressing skepticism about the accuracy of his method—phone surveys—to measure illegal or clandestine behavior.

Both perspectives help to illuminate the dimensions of Fighting Back, as well as the continuing debate on its merits. This debate—whose outcome almost certainly will influence future community-based substance abuse initiatives—revolves around three distinct but intertwined issues: the goals of the program, the way it was evaluated, and midcourse changes in program direction.

### The Original Goals of the Program

The Foundation's 1989 call for proposals was explicit on performance expectations, calling for

- A measurable and sustained reduction in the initiation of drug and alcohol use among children and adolescents

- A reduction in drug- and alcohol-related deaths and injuries, especially among children, adolescents, and young adults
- A decline in the prevalence of health problems related to or exacerbated by drug and alcohol abuse
- A reduction in on-the-job problems and injuries related to substance abuse
- A reduction in drug-related crime

Beyond these specific performance expectations, Fighting Back had some larger goals, according to the program's architects, Hearn and Jellinek. Hearn contends that Fighting Back from the very beginning was an "efficacy trial," to test whether broad-based community efforts *could* make a dent in substance abuse. Jellinek adds that its larger purpose was to challenge public despair over substance abuse and restore a sense of optimism to communities struggling with its consequences and to the nation as a whole.

### The Evaluation

In a program surrounded by controversy, the most contentious issue of all concerns the evaluation. Critics argue that the evaluation was flawed in a number of key respects:

- First, it looked at the wrong things. In noting that Fighting Back was an "efficacy" trial, Hearn says Saxe's survey solely measured "effectiveness," which is something different. "We were asking, Can it be done?" she said. "We weren't asking, Can it be done in six different places?" Jellinek, meanwhile, argues that the evaluation failed to capture the larger goals of restoring optimism and confidence at the community level. He asserts that post–Fighting Back, drug use in the United States has gone down across the board, including at Fighting Back test sites; public confidence has gone up; and community coalitions built under Fighting Back continue to address substance abuse in an integrated fashion. "So the irony is we accomplished our goals, but the evaluation says it didn't work," Jellinek says.

- Second, the methodology—a telephone survey—was flawed. Critics say that it's laughable to think that people will reveal whether they use drugs to an interviewer on the other end of a telephone.

- Third, the survey sample was tainted. Hearn notes that the federal Center for Substance Abuse Prevention poured $375 million into 251 community partnerships patterned after Fighting Back, some of them in Fighting Back communities. With similar activities under different auspices going on in both treatment and some comparison sites, Hearn questioned whether the evaluation could adequately tease out Fighting Back's influences from those of other forces in the community.

- Fourth, the evaluation was underfunded. Critics charge that changing evaluators in midstream resulted in the loss of roughly $4.6 million of the original $11.5 million allocated to measure Fighting Back results. Though Saxe says he and program officers at the Foundation pushed for additional funding, in the end he was told to make do.

Responding to these criticisms, James Knickman, the Foundation's vice president for research and evaluation, characterizes the arguments as little more than Monday morning quarterbacking. He argues that

- The call for proposals was unequivocal in stating that measurable change in the Fighting Back communities was the program's objective. Everyone agreed the Foundation had to have bottom-line numbers. Moreover, he adds, for an overall investment of $88 million, it was reasonable to expect tangible results.

- The Foundation's program officers and Saxe signed off on the phone survey methodology as a commonly used tool in substance abuse research, even while acknowledging it to be a "fallible, second-best measure." In fact, the rates measured from the telephone survey tracked those estimated in various national surveys using other data collection methods, offering support for the validity of the telephone survey methodology.

- The concern about a tainted sample doesn't hold up. Three comparison sites were studied for each Fighting Back site and even when "contaminated" sites were accounted for, no program impact was detected.

- The evaluation, both initially and subsequently, was amply funded.

### Changes in Program Direction

Managerial upheaval was not limited to the evaluation. In 1996 the Foundation transferred the National Program Office from Vanderbilt University to Join Together, an organization at the Boston University School of Public Health that supports community-based efforts to combat substance abuse. David Rosenbloom, who heads Join Together, became the national program director.

Rosenbloom immediately abandoned the governance structure of broad-based community coalitions so explicitly laid out in the Fighting Back call for proposals. At the same time, he curtailed the freedom of Fighting Back communities to pursue homegrown interventions, emphasizing the development of services to treat and deter substance abuse. In short, Fighting Back's operating strategy was completely revamped halfway through the experiment. Grantees say the program's emphasis changed dramatically under Rosenbloom, and sites redirected their projects accordingly, abandoning efforts that could not quickly produce measurable results. Also at this juncture, the Foundation terminated funding for six of the original fourteen sites.

—ɯ— **Ideal Meets Reality: The Experiences of Worcester, Massachusetts, and Vallejo, California**

Anyone who has participated in his or her community—whether as church volunteer, sewer commissioner, block cleanup captain, or PTA mom—knows how hard it is to achieve consensus and how late the meetings can run, even among people who share a common vision. The people reading the Fighting Back call for proposals were veterans of such community efforts. Some mused about the size of the conference room they were going to need to assemble the Fighting Back team. Others, knowing of existing conflicts within the group defined by The Robert Wood Johnson Foundation, wondered how consensus could ever be reached on something as polarized as substance abuse.

Yet 331 communities applied for Fighting Back grants. The Foundation had projected a maximum of 125 applications, based on eligibility criteria that limited the program to midsize cities with populations between 100,000 and 250,000. According to Kay Sherwood, author of a case study on the Fighting Back evaluation, staff members at the Foundation took the high volume of applicants "as a sign that they had tapped a reservoir of interest and concern at the community level about drug use and abuse."[3]

Worcester, Massachusetts, and Vallejo, California, were among the fourteen midsize cities selected to test the Foundation's assumptions. Both communities entered the arena of Fighting Back in 1990 buoyed by success in winning the grants. Neither city is accustomed to national attention. Worcester lives in the shadow of Boston, an hour's drive to the east, and Vallejo is underdog to San Francisco, an hour's drive to the southwest. In this modest context, landing $3.2 million from an East Coast philanthropy was front-page news.

But the two communities would end up very differently in the anecdotal history of Fighting Back. When Fighting Back insiders want to showcase the program's achievements, they hold up Vallejo. For failures, they point to Worcester. What's remarkable, however, is how similarly the people of Vallejo and the people of Worcester articulate the lessons they learned in field-testing the Foundation's theories.

Both communities had grappled with substance abuse before Fighting Back came on the scene. Vallejo, a city of 119,000 that grew up around the former navy shipyard at Mare Island, had a long history of alcohol problems and a growing problem with "crank," or methamphetamine, addiction. Worcester, a manufacturing city of 173,000, was worried about heroin, in addition to alcohol. A spike in hepatitis B cases in Worcester in the mid-1980s, which the federal Centers for Disease Control and Prevention attributed to addicts sharing contaminated needles, heightened public alarm about the city's drug problem.

But leaders in both cities said the size of the Fighting Back grant—$3 million—was also a powerful lure, given the bleak economic conditions at the time. National unemployment was moving up, tax revenues were down, and municipal budgets were under strain.

"You've got to understand how bad that recession was and how much it affected our thinking about the drug problem and about Fighting Back," says Lieutenant Alexander Donoghue, a thirty-three-year veteran of the Worcester Police Department, much of his career spent on drug-related crime. Donoghue was an early and enthusiastic participant in Worcester Fights Back, grateful, he says, for the prospect of community-wide help with a problem he knew police couldn't solve alone.

"This department had laid off fifty officers, which it had never done in its history," Donoghue recalls. "Teachers were being laid off. Real estate prices were plummeting, and people were literally walking away from income real estate that they had bought high. We had two hundred to three hundred triple-deckers"—classic New England wood frame housing with three apartments stacked one atop the other—"vacant, which are like magnets to the drug trade." He explains, "It was an ugly scene, and here comes a chance to bring in $3 million in outside money when our budgets were being slashed to nothing."

The lead agency on Worcester's application was the United Way of Central Massachusetts. Eric Buch, now the organization's president, was point man on the application. Reading the Fighting Back call for proposals, he thought the model was "very diverse," calling for broad-based action on a bewildering number of fronts. But the level of detail persuaded him that The Robert Wood Johnson Foundation had "done its homework."

"We were told that in order to make a serious effort against a very entrenched problem we had to show involvement in virtually every sector of the community," Buch recalls. "From a theoretical standpoint, it made sense, and since we did not come from the substance abuse field we trusted the people who designed the program."

One section of the call for proposals laid out state-of-the-art public health methodology for ameliorating harm, including public awareness campaigns, expanded treatment options, and prevention education for children and youth. Buch and others on Worcester's organizing committee thought this made sense as well. Indeed, if Fighting Back had been a clear-cut health initiative—say, immunizing babies against the threat of infectious disease—results of the sort detailed in the call for proposals likely would have been achieved. The evil—disease—is unequivocal, and there is public consensus that babies are worth protecting. There is also strong science on the safety and efficacy of vaccine, as well as established and consistent government policy to provide a framework for effective community action.

But Fighting Back had none of these assets, veterans of the experiment say. Federal and state policies on substance abuse were fragmented and discordant, as Foundation staff learned from their own research. Addiction science was weak at the inception of Fighting Back, and the impact of popular prevention models, such as DARE, was in dispute. Public opinion ranged widely as to cause and responsibility for alcohol and drug addiction, and the concept of substance abuse as a "public health" problem was largely unknown.

It made for a very confusing conversation around the task force table as community leaders, addiction specialists, recovering addicts, neighborhood representatives, police, parents, politicians, clergy, schoolteachers, and business owners struggled to find a common language by which to identify the "evil" and then figure out how to go after it.

Al Donoghue, the Worcester police lieutenant who was so enthusiastic at the outset, found his interest waning. From a regular attendee at task force meetings, he dropped to every other meeting, then every third.

"Quite frankly, I began to feel I was out of my element," he recalled in an interview at police headquarters. "They had all these buzzwords, like a whole insider language." Donoghue rummaged through his desk for an illustration, pulling out an old report of the local project, Worcester Fights Back. "'A longitudinal study of a cohort of sixth graders,'" he read. "The 'disease model of drug addiction . . .' I didn't know what the hell they were talking about after a while."

Language and definitional disputes turned out to be rampant in Fighting Back, even within subgroups of the larger coalitions mandated by the program. Recovering addicts, for example, disagree on the definition of alcohol abuse versus alcoholism, or whether you can call yourself "clean and sober" if you're on legitimately prescribed medication, or whether crack is more dangerous than methamphetamine, according to Jeannie Villarreal, a former crack addict and Fighting Back worker in Vallejo. Villarreal's Fighting Back assignment has been to organize recovering drug users into mutually supportive networks that might also be forces for community education and outreach.

"We are mostly twelve-step people; but we are starting to get some faith-based recovering addicts, and we are also trying to get some methadone people," Villarreal says. "But that's going to be controversial because a lot of the twelve-steppers don't like the idea of substituting one drug for another. They don't consider the methadone users 'clean.'" The same prejudice exists, she and others in the recovery community say, against people with underlying psychiatric conditions whose slide into addiction might well have been the result of self-medicating. Will recovery support groups accept them if they are now taking psychotropic medication? Villarreal is not sure. And this was the state of things in Fighting Back's flagship community in late 2002.

Which is not to say that Vallejo, Worcester, and the twelve other Fighting Back alliances failed to alter the conversation around drugs and alcohol in their communities or add resources that didn't exist before. They did. But none of them were able to make their communities speak with one voice about substance abuse. The difficulty of changing attitudes and building consensus was underestimated not only by the Foundation but also by Fighting Back community leaders who tried to galvanize community action. Worcester had an immediate marketing problem with the Foundation's decision to lump alcohol *abuse* and illegal drug *use* under the substance abuse/public health problem umbrella as if they were twin evils.

This was not the original concept of Fighting Back; Foundation trustees had asked for an antidrug program. But early in the planning process, the task forces on alcohol and drugs were merged, according to Ruby Hearn, and discussion began to focus on their similarities. In the culture of the health-oriented Foundation, it was easy to see them as chronic illnesses requiring treatment and support. There was also clinical evidence to support this, as many drug addicts also abuse alcohol and vice versa.

But it was also a numbers issue, according to David Rosenbloom, Fighting Back's national program director. Alcohol abuse is far more prevalent than illegal drug use in the United States. Estimates, based on the definition of abuse, range widely (the Fighting Back call for proposals said 10 percent of Americans abuse alcohol,[4] but other studies put that number as high as 25 percent[5]). As a clandestine activity, illegal drug use is harder to measure, but it is generally agreed to represent a small fraction of the substance abuse problem. So including alcohol abuse made broad-based community action more likely.

Perhaps an early warning of the definitional confusion that would play out in the field and of the difficulty in selling a combined assault on illegal drugs and alcohol was the lack of apples-to-apples comparative data in Fighting Back's call for proposals. Only when it came to projected costs to society was the call for proposals able to make a direct relationship between alcohol and illegal drug use: of $229 billion expected in 1990, $136 billion would be due to alcohol abuse, $76 billion to illegal drug abuse, and $17 billion to intravenous drug–related AIDS.

In Worcester, public feeling against illegal drug use was high, but the reaction to alcohol was more equivocal. Fighting Back workers attributed this not only to the fact that one was illegal while the other was legal but to cultural norms as well. For starters, business and community leaders routinely served alcohol at fundraisers and professional gatherings. And taverns, liquor stores, and beer wholesalers were part of the city's business infrastructure. So while it was relatively easy to get consensus on action against illegal drug use, alcohol was a more complicated conversation.

"There were some attempts to lobby the city council about liquor licenses, but they were few and far between," says Jack Bonina, a social worker who was on the paid staff of Worcester Fights Back. "The drug issue was easier to get people organized around because it brings crime, prostitution, violence, plus the medical issues: AIDS, HIV, all of that. Alcohol is a much harder sell. You end up looking like a fringe person railing against the societal mainstream. This was the case not only in the corporate community but also in the neighborhoods."

Race and class issues also interfered with consensus in Fighting Back. Jewel Fink, a Vallejo school official, encountered the race factor when it became her job to announce a substance abuse prevention minigrants program for Vallejo neighborhoods. At the time, Fink was the Vallejo City Unified School District's liaison to the local project, the Fighting Back Partnership.

"I knew I was in trouble when I walked into the room and there were the white people in the front seats, the African Americans on one side, the Filipinos on the other side, and the Mexicans in the back," recalls Fink, who runs the Vallejo school system's substance abuse and pregnancy prevention programs. "I was supposed to be running a workshop on how to apply for the grants and how they were going to be judged on a merit basis. But the people in the room were really stuck on this idea that they were owed a share of the money. Then one of the Latinos in the back stood up and said, 'Why should everyone get the same money? Everyone knows the Filipinos are rich and the blacks get everything, and we're the losers every time.' Basically, he wanted more than the others got, and we hadn't even talked about anything that the money would be used for."

For Fink, that workshop crystallized a perspective of community that was not the Fighting Back ideal but might be the only way to get diverse constituencies on board. People had their own idea of what constituted community, and edicts from the Fighting Back citizens' task force weren't likely to change that.

Worcester also had an early experience underscoring the divisions among constituencies that defeated collective action. The blowup came on the very day that Worcester was celebrating its selection as a Fighting Back city. An announcement party was organized at Mechanics Hall, an elegant nineteenth-century brick building on Main Street that is an iconic gathering spot for civic celebration. Everyone who had participated in the planning process and nearly two hundred community leaders whose organizations had contributed letters of support were invited to attend. "I think it was the last time all of us ever got together happily in one room," says Donald Chamberlayne, a Worcester Police Department crime analyst who was the Worcester project's in-house research and data specialist.

The meeting, Chamberlayne and others say, kicked off with the usual celebratory speeches. Then Lois Green, who chaired United Way of Central Massachusetts at the time, stood to read a list of about thirty people who would serve on the initiative's steering committee. It was a blue-ribbon list, representing all of the municipal partners the Fighting Back call for proposals had mandated, as well as a cross section of community leaders. But it was weighted toward those with the heft to push through institutional change.

A minister representing Hispanic residents in whose impoverished neighborhoods much of the visible drug activity took place stood to ask whether nominations to the steering committee would be accepted from the floor. She was told no, the membership was set. Hearing that, the minister turned and marched out of the hall, trailed by several other Hispanic representatives. It was a startlingly discordant moment in what should have been a cheerful gathering. But in retrospect, says Chamberlayne, it was a "a symbol of the rift that was never quite fixable."

The minister's action underscored perceptual issues that would be the source of continuing tension in Fighting Back efforts to craft action plans that could be sold community-wide. If Fighting Back was an anti–substance abuse initiative, then shouldn't those most burdened by substance abuse have a strong voice in its deployment? But who was most burdened? Using data gathered from phone surveys of Fighting Back communities, Saxe, the program's evaluator, concluded that although *visible* drug activity— manifested by drunks, drug dealers, crime—is more prevalent in poor neighborhoods, actual drug use varies little from neighborhood to neighborhood.[6]

The fact is that by taking on substance abuse as a civic issue, Fighting Back leaders and field workers were up against attitudes heavily freighted with moral judgments, fear, and biases that flowed from individual perception and personal experience with drug and alcohol abuse. This made the Foundation's labeling of substance abuse as a "public health problem" and addiction as "chronic illness" a particularly hard sell in neighborhoods where the detritus of the drug trade—condoms, dirty needles—litters the sidewalks and residents live in fear of reprisal from drug dealers.

Juan Gonzalez is a case in point. A stalwart of Vallejo's Fighting Back project, he nevertheless flashes anger at the notion of addicts being "sick" people in need of help. For him, Fighting Back was literally that: turning the tables on the drug dealers who terrorized his family. "If it wasn't for Fighting Back, I'd probably be in jail myself, because I was going to hurt somebody," he says.

Gonzalez lives with his wife and two daughters on Coronel Avenue, a neighborhood of modest stucco homes. An immigrant from a poor village in Mexico, Gonzalez works double shifts as a waiter in a San Francisco hotel to provide a safe home for his family. Coronel Avenue was such a place until the drug dealers moved in next door.

In contrast to the Gonzalez's tidy property with its rose beds and burbling fountain, the "drug house" is barely visible behind overgrown shrubbery and a front yard strewn with junk. The family's ordeal began after a beer and drug party involving dozens of young men spilled over into the Gonzalez yard and Juan Gonzalez stepped out to confront them.

"They laughed in my face," Gonzalez remembers. Soon, the parties were every-night occurrences. Intoxicated men and women rampaged through yards up and down the street. They urinated on the Gonzalez flower beds, dumped beer cans and drug paraphernalia on the lawn, and on several occasions went so far as to stand at the windows and expose themselves to Gonzalez's young daughters.

"It wasn't just us; it was the whole neighborhood," Gonzalez recounts. "Everyone on the street had their tires slashed. We called them the bat boys, because they carried baseball bats to intimidate people."

For protection, Gonzalez and his wife took to sleeping on the floor of the kitchen, which had a window overlooking the front yard. This lasted for more than a year. One day, a Fighting Back representative knocked at Gonzalez's door, saying he'd heard from police contacts that there had been drug trouble in the neighborhood.

"I told him the whole story," says Gonzalez. "I told him I was calling the police five times a day without response. I told him I was desperate and that my girls were scared. He sent a letter to Lieutenant [Reginald] Garcia"—the police department liaison to Fighting Back—"and Lieutenant Garcia came over to see me."

It was the beginning of a coordinated effort with the police department to restore a sense of safety to the neighborhood. With Fighting Back's help, residents formed neighborhood patrols, developed cooperative relationships with police, and learned to use city services—housing code enforcement, for example—to discipline negligent landlords. Barbara Gaddies, a volunteer who lives in a predominantly African American neighborhood known as the Crest, said that these tactics, taught by Fighting Back organizers, also helped rid her street of drug dealers.

## —⟋⟍— Restructuring the Program

Vallejo's strategy of targeting interventions to meet specific needs articulated by specific communities was that city's way of reconciling the early mandates of Fighting Back with the political realities of community action. These realities, mirrored in feedback from other Fighting Back communities, led to The Robert Wood Johnson Foundation's 1996 overhaul of the program. The desired results—measurable declines in alcohol and drug use—had not been achieved, and program staff members argued for more time as well as for new leadership. With Rosenbloom at the helm and a revamped field strategy in place, the Foundation agreed to allocate $20.8 million over five years to eight of the fourteen original test sites.[7]

Under Rosenbloom, Fighting Back no longer required participating cities to maintain the broad community task force specified in the original proposal. In a December 1996 memorandum to the renewed sites, Rosenbloom reviewed the lessons of the experiment's first seven years: "Each of our communities has developed its own approach and structure, and some of them differ markedly from the original ideas about the components of the program. Governance structures are quite varied; some sites target only parts of the community; and the notion of a comprehensive single community-wide system of prevention and treatment has never been fully developed."

Rosenbloom told the sites to choose their own form of governance. "The key here is a structure that works for your community and for the goals you have identified," he wrote in the memorandum. At the same time, however, he sharply curtailed the freedom that sites had enjoyed to pick their own targets and intervention strategies, and narrowed their options. Now sites were encouraged to concentrate their efforts on alcohol or on a specific drug rather than on all drug and alcohol problems, as in the first phase of Fighting Back. No site would get money unless it submitted a three-year strategic plan stating clearly "how the projects will make measurable improvements in specific agreed-upon outcome measures in key neighborhoods or population groups," Rosenbloom's memorandum stated. "Success in achieving these outcome objectives will be required to obtain funding for the remaining two years."

Jane Callahan, director of the Vallejo project at the time and now director of the Community Anti-Drug Coalition Institute, said the discipline imposed by Rosenbloom made the difference in her community's ability to make inroads against substance abuse.

"All of a sudden, we got clear on what the hell Fighting Back was all about," she says. "Before, it was just all over the map. Someone would come to a meeting and bang the table and say we need parenting programs, and the next week we would dutifully start a parenting program. We thought that was what we were supposed to do: be responsive to our constituents."

Freed from the unwieldy organizational structure of the original program and newly empowered to tailor programs to specific constituencies, Vallejo launched school-based programs that, among other things, give classroom teachers training in substance abuse issues and provide mentors to at-risk middle school students. Vallejo Fighting Back also helped establish the Solano County Drug Court, instituted addiction treatment in county jails, and collaborated with Kaiser Permanente on expanding substance abuse treatment services to recipients of Medicaid (called "Medi-Cal" in California). Youth Partnership, the program that helped young James leave gang life, also came into existence during this time, as did the Vallejo Neighborhood Revitalization program, from which Juan Gonzalez and his family benefited.

Callahan is proud of these accomplishments but regrets the time lost before Fighting Back found its focus. "The fact is, we spent the first six years in trial and error, spinning our wheels," Callahan says. "The Foundation kept talking numerator and denominator to prove results, and I didn't have a clue. What I wish I would have learned from the beginning was true strategic planning."

Vallejo got a second chance to achieve its goals, but Worcester did not. It was one of the six original Fighting Back sites dropped from the program. Rather than feeling slighted, Worcester reacted with relief. Project leaders do not dispute that their effort had foundered. In part, they blame an early project manager who played constituencies off against one another and the local task force against national program leaders. The manager was replaced; but hard feelings and mistrust had set in, and subsequent managers were unable to recover the unity of the planning phase.

"Fighting Back did a lot of damage," says Patsy Lewis, executive director of the Worcester Community Action Council and a member of Worcester Fights Back's steering committee. She regrets that the city did not have the self-confidence to assert its own style of community initiative but instead squandered time, money, and energy in "i-dotting and t-crossing" to comply with Foundation mandates.

"There were connections in this city between business and schools and communities that we could have built on," Lewis says. "But the model imposed on us was so rigid. We had to gather up specified elements of the community that weren't necessarily natural allies to this effort. The call for proposals did not allow Worcester to be Worcester."

Jill Dagilis, city hall's delegate to the Fighting Back coalition, concurs. "It was such a false expectation that you could put everyone around a table and just go," she says. "Fighting Back was so discouraging—we haven't wanted to work together on that scope of citywide initiative since. People still socialize and network, but on a particular project, they only want to work with a couple of agencies, reverting to traditional liaisons."

## —ɯ— Conclusion

These are some headlines that appeared as Fighting Back wrapped up:

- "Suspicious House Fire Kills 6; Mother, Five Children Die . . . Neighbors say fatal blaze was retaliation for stand against drug dealing" (*The Baltimore Sun,* June 17, 2002).

- "Crack Is . . . Back? In Williamsburg, hipsters are taking eighties revivalism to a whole other level" (*New York Magazine,* Nov. 18, 2002).

- "Doctors to Pay Tab for New Drug Fight: Bush team plans to double licensing fees for physicians, pharmacies and manufacturers to combat the abuse of prescription drugs" (*The Los Angeles Times,* Feb. 11, 2003, front page).

Might these suggest an answer to Steven Schroeder's question "Why all the heat?" The people who worked for twelve years to implement Fighting Back's precepts would say "Yes!" More than any flaws in program design, implementation, or evaluative methodology, it was the arena in which The Robert Wood Johnson Foundation chose to do battle that accounts for the intensity of feeling at every level of Fighting Back.

The Foundation chose to define substance abuse as a chronic illness. It then packaged Fighting Back as a public health initiative, lumping together alcohol abuse and illegal drug use and calling on communities to band together against these twin ills. It sought to join the efforts of traditional players in the substance abuse field—police, medical professionals, and addiction specialists—with school and civic officials, business leaders, neighborhood groups, and recovering addicts. And it commissioned a quantitative evaluation that hewed closely to the standards of the hard sciences.

But substance abuse is messier than that, as the people who carried out the program quickly learned. They realized, as the headlines remind us, that substance abuse is not just a disease but a danger. It is also a moving target, ebbing for a time only to return in unexpected fashion. Crack, for example, was chiefly a scourge of poor, inner-city, and predominantly African American neighborhoods in the 1980s. In 2002 a *New York Magazine* article reported on use by mostly white, elite, club-hopping types out for kicks.[8]

Defining substance abuse as a chronic illness—an area in which the Foundation had been working for years—probably made Fighting Back easier for the Foundation to understand and to fund. But it couldn't be sold at the community level. Drunk drivers were killing people. Drug dealers were terrorizing neighborhoods. Among Fighting Back activists were people who had lost children to drug and alcohol addiction or who had struggled with it themselves. They knew the damaging ripple effects on family members, coworkers, and communities. To them, substance abuse was not simply a chronic illness like asthma or diabetes; it was a public menace.

Lumping alcohol and illegal drugs into a single initiative without acknowledging their social distinctions created another problem. Medically, this makes sense; drugs and alcohol are both addictive, and many substance abusers have poly-addictions. But those fighting illegal drugs and those fighting alcohol abuse were fighting different battles. As in the tragic case of the Baltimore mother and her children, killed in retaliation for antidrug activism, drugs raise questions of personal safety: of gun violence, of junkies on the stoop, of prostitutes in the alleyways. Alcohol abuse raises other issues—brawls, drunk driving—but not (to the same extent) the issues of violent crime and neighborhood deterioration.

All this made it difficult to hold the community coalitions together. And they didn't hold. In the end, no Fighting Back project was able to sustain the Foundation-prescribed task force. All of them retreated to smaller alliances of people joined by common interest à la Juan Gonzalez's neighborhood improvement group. At Fighting Back's final meeting in March 2003, Bonita Grubbs of New Haven, Connecticut, called the required task forces "window dressing" approaches to the idea of broad-based community action, an opinion seconded by many others.

Finally, there is the Fighting Back evaluation, once again reflecting The Robert Wood Johnson Foundation's hard-science orientation of the 1980s. Much has changed since then. The Foundation has commissioned qualitative and descriptive evaluations to better capture lessons from its growing portfolio of social change initiatives. At Fighting Back's inception, however, the quantitative approach to measuring success ruled.

Most Fighting Back grantees heard the evaluation's "no measurable impact" verdict for the first time at the March 2003 meeting. Remarkably, for all the heat the evaluation has generated among Fighting Back's national leaders, those who carried out the experiment seem neither impressed nor discouraged by the findings.

"I'm not an evaluation expert. I'm just a member of a community who worked on this for twelve years," said Peter MacDougall, a retired community college president in Santa Barbara, California. "But I have to say all these issues at the top created only mild ripples in the local community. Once we had our plan, that was our project and that's what we pursued. . . . Our day-to-day decision making was really focused on what can work here and what can we do to make it work better."

The Santa Barbara project resisted pressure from the National Program Office to go community-wide, focusing instead on school-age youngsters, in the belief that they would benefit most from Fighting Back interventions. The work continues today; Santa Barbara's is one of the Fighting Back projects still active at the end of Robert Wood Johnson Foundation funding. It's not surprising, given the project's narrow focus, that community-wide reductions in substance abuse could not be measured by the evaluation. But that in no way diminishes Santa Barbara's sense that Fighting Back resulted in sustainable improvements.

William Cirone, superintendent of schools in Santa Barbara County, counts one success as getting his community "past denial to awareness." He quipped that his schools probably registered higher now in statistical measures of substance abuse because of new programs to get the problem out in the open, identify troubled students, and get them help. Jewel Fink of the Vallejo, California, project said essentially the same thing: because Vallejo schools now aim to get youngsters into treatment while keeping them in school, they consistently look worse on statistical reports than a neighboring school district with a zero-tolerance policy.

This was the tenor of the conversation at Fighting Back's final gathering. The accounts of triumphs and setbacks, false starts and unexpected dividends filled two days in a conference room, and continued after hours. The participants talked candidly about the frustration of working against an age-old problem that, as recent headlines demonstrate, persists for all the reasons the nascent science of addiction has given us: environmental factors, social pressures, and, more recently, brain chemistry. The Fighting Back veterans uniformly describe their experiences as two steps forward, one step back. Quantifying success was a struggle for all of them, except on the most idiosyncratic level. An example is the Gallup project, which focused only on alcohol abuse and was not part of the national evaluation. Nevertheless, executive director Raymond Daw said his task force strove to measure progress via a number of local indicators, one of them being winter exposure deaths among the acutely intoxicated on and around the Indian reservations of Northwest New Mexico. These dropped from 270 annually to 86—a statistic that Daw says means a great deal to the citizens who worked on education, treatment, and prevention programs. However, Daw counts as an equally important indicator of progress that Native Americans now sit on municipal committees previously controlled by whites. Is that a Fighting Back success? In a community where the historical definition of substance abuse was "drunk Indians," it is indeed.

As is the rescue of young James from the Vallejo street gang, even if the specific cause and effect remain elusive. James was quick to credit Fighting Back at the beginning of our conversation. But even he wrestles with questions about why he did what he did and why things turned out OK when they might not for someone else.

"I can't really say what it was specifically that made me go another way," he muses as we say good-bye. "I guess it was good my sister took me to Youth Partnership. And we had some mentors there who had done time at San Quentin for drug dealing; so they could tell us what it was really like, and that was scary."

He packs up some sample posters he'd brought to our interview; they feature the winners of an anti-drug-and-alcohol art contest organized by James and other youth volunteers in city schools each year.

"Whatever," he shrugs, "I'm glad I'm where I'm at now."

## Notes

1. Jellinek, P. S., and Hearn, R. P. "Fighting Drug Abuse at the Local Level." *Issues in Science and Technology* (National Academy of Sciences), 1991, *7*(4).
2. This Gallup, New Mexico, program is examined in Brodeur, P. "Combating Alcohol Abuse in Northwestern New Mexico: Gallup's Fighting Back and Healthy Nations Programs." In *To Improve Health and Health Care, Vol. VI: The Robert Wood Johnson Foundation Anthology.* San Francisco: Jossey-Bass, 2003.

3. Sherwood, K. E. *Evaluation of Fighting Back.* (Unpublished). The Robert Wood Johnson Foundation, 2002.

4. *Call for Proposals, Fighting Back: Community Initiative to Reduce Demand for Illegal Drugs and Alcohol.* The Robert Wood Johnson Foundation, 1989.

5. *Reducing Risky Drinking: A Report on Early Identification and Management of Alcohol Problems Through Screening and Brief Intervention.* Alcohol Research Center, University of Connecticut Health Center, 1996.

6. Saxe, L., and others. "The Visibility of Illicit Drugs: Implications for Community-Based Drug Control Strategies." *American Journal of Public Health,* 2002, *91*(12), 1987–1994.

7. The eight sites were New Haven, Little Rock, San Antonio, Kansas City, Santa Barbara, Vallejo, Washington, D.C., and Newark.

8. *New York Magazine,* Nov. 18, 2002.

# 2

# Join Together and CADCA

## Backing Up the Front Line

*Paul Jellinek and Renie Schapiro*

### Editors' Introduction

In 1989, a time when the nation was in the midst of an anguishing drug crisis, the Foundation launched the Fighting Back program to support anti–substance abuse coalitions in fourteen communities throughout the nation. Irene Wielawski examines this program in the preceding chapter. Community coalitions—which comprise community leaders, substance abuse treatment providers, law enforcement agencies, school systems, youth organizations, citizens, and advocates—were seen at the time as crucial to mobilizing local activity to decrease the use of drugs and alcohol. Even before Fighting Back was up and running, the U.S. government adopted the model and funded 251 community anti–substance abuse coalitions.

The creation of so many community coalitions to fight substance abuse was new, difficult, and important enough to justify the Foundation's spending additional money to try to make sure they succeeded. So the Foundation provided funding for two organizations—Join Together in 1991 and Community Anti-Drug Coalitions of America, or CADCA, in 1992—to nurture the coalitions and provide them with technical support. While technical support is a common element of Foundation strategy, this case was atypical in that *two* technical support organizations were funded, and they provided assistance to coalitions outside of the Foundation's Fighting Back program as well.

As the authors of this chapter—Paul Jellinek, a former vice president of The Robert Wood Johnson Foundation who was involved in the development and monitoring of grants that supported community coalitions, and Renie Schapiro, a freelance writer and consultant to the Foundation who has written extensively on the subject of substance abuse—recount, Join Together and CADCA offered substantially different approaches to technical support. CADCA is a membership organization that, in addition to providing technical assistance, acts as a trade organization in Washington, D.C. Join Together complements its one-on-one technical support with an ambitious policy analysis and publication agenda and a highly regarded Web site that directs readers to a large array of resources related to substance abuse.

This year's *Anthology* contains three chapters on programs dealing with community-based coalitions.[1] None of the programs turned out to be effective in solving the problems they were set up to address—substance abuse and escalating health care costs. This may mean that the problems are too endemic to be solved at the community level or by community coalitions, that the community coalition model doesn't work, or that the model has not been implemented well. As the authors of all three chapters note, community coalitions are messy and, to an extent, challenge human nature by requiring people with few common interests to collaborate. Given the difficulties, it is not surprising Jellinek and Schapiro suggest that if community coalitions are to succeed, they will need a healthy dose of technical support.

---

1. This chapter; Chapter One; and Chapter Three, which has a section on the Community Programs for Affordable Health Care initiative.

—ᴡ— **B**y the time Susan Weed was appointed director of the City of Chicago Office of Substance Abuse Policy in November 1994, the drug crisis was no longer on the cover of the nation's news weeklies, as it had been in the mid-1980s, when crack burst upon the national scene and Len Bias, the promising young basketball star at the University of Maryland, died a widely publicized death from a cocaine overdose. The president no longer talked about drugs as a national priority—if at all—and William Bennett, the nation's first drug czar, had long since moved on to other, greener policy pastures.

But in the streets of Chicago, as in many other neighborhoods and communities all over the country, the crisis was far from over. "It was the violence that people were most concerned about," Weed recalls. "There was a lot of violence associated with the sale and trafficking of drugs. It was just one drive-by shooting after another. That really scared people and made it difficult for them to see substance abuse as anything other than a law enforcement issue."

Weed, who came from the city's health department, saw the issue in terms other than law enforcement. "Mayor Daley understood that law enforcement had a very important role to play, but in the end you had to do something about demand," Weed says. "And that was a public health issue."

Defining substance abuse as a public health issue sounds simple enough. Actually implementing an effective public health strategy turns out to be a very tall order indeed. It means finding ways to prevent large numbers of people throughout the community—especially young people—from becoming involved in substance abuse in the first place. It means intervening early with counseling and other support if they do get involved. It means getting people into more intensive treatment if early intervention has failed and they've become seriously involved. And it means providing the full range of aftercare and support they need to get their lives back together if and when they've successfully completed treatment.

Each of these elements of the strategy, in turn, is fraught with complexity. For instance, convincing an already overburdened urban school system to adopt a model substance abuse prevention curriculum is hard enough. But hard as it is, a new prevention curriculum by itself isn't likely to have much impact if the neighborhoods the students return to after school are plastered with alcohol and cigarette billboards; if forty-ounce cans of malt liquor are freely sold to minors at the neighborhood corner stores; if there is little for young people to do after school other than to hang out on the streets with the wrong kinds of role models. Similarly, more treatment by itself probably won't make much of a difference if those individuals who do successfully complete treatment are shunned by the community and can't find a decent job or a place to live.

Weed quickly realized that implementing an effective public health strategy that would begin to get at the roots of Chicago's substance abuse problem would require the active engagement and collaboration of a host of public agencies, community organizations, and neighborhood residents, many of whom hadn't worked together before or, if they had, didn't necessarily trust one another.

Moreover, Weed says, many of them didn't see substance abuse as their responsibility. "With the exception of law enforcement, agencies we recruited would readily acknowledge that substance abuse was a big problem, and, please, let them know what they could do," she said. "But none of them owned it. The City of Chicago government has about fifty separate departments. We were able to identify substance abuse issues that each one should be grappling with. But while they—and private organizations as well—would acknowledge their part of the problem, it was not their main mission. And when it comes to allocating human and financial resources, they go to those activities central to their mission."

In any community, pulling such a broad-based collaborative effort together and convincing all the players to give substance abuse the high priority it warranted would have been a daunting challenge. In a city the size and complexity of Chicago—where at that time, Weed says, it was estimated that more than half a million people had a serious substance abuse problem—it was almost overwhelming.

## —⚏— Join Together

Shortly after Weed became the director of Chicago's Office of Substance Abuse Policy, she heard of Join Together, a national organization funded by The Robert Wood Johnson Foundation to support local substance abuse initiatives. "One of my staff members found Join Together," Weed recalls. "She told me about their fellowship program, and she said I should apply. So I did, and I was accepted."

The fellowship, one of Join Together's signature programs, eventually supported and connected more than two hundred individuals throughout the nation who played key leadership roles in addressing substance abuse in their communities—elected officials, citizen activists, business executives, health professionals, educators, police officers, substance abuse professionals, judges, union leaders, journalists, and many others.

"It was wonderful," Weed says. "We learned so much from the program—and from each other. I always came back from the meetings with new ideas, new people to partner with, new sources of funding. I've interacted with other fellows from the program for many, many reasons since then. For instance, when we were looking to start a residential program for families with substance abuse problems here in Chicago, I was able to identify four or five other places around the country that had already done it. So we didn't have to start from scratch."

She adds, "And then there was the moral support. That was really very important: just knowing there were other people out there coping with the same problems. And the staff at Join Together was always there for me. They sent e-mails; they made phone calls. I felt like we were not alone."

It was precisely this notion—that local leaders like Susan Weed, who were grappling with the drug crisis on the front lines of America's cities and towns, should not be out there on their own—that gave rise to Join Together in the first place. The idea for Join Together first came up during a train ride on a rainy November evening in 1990. Ruby Hearn, then a vice president at The Robert Wood Johnson Foundation, and Paul Jellinek, then a senior program officer at the Foundation, were on the Metroliner from Washington, D.C., back to the Foundation's offices in New Jersey. They had just spent two days at a conference convened by President George H. W. Bush's Drug Advisory Council that had brought together hundreds of representatives from local substance abuse initiatives from all over the country, including a number of grantees from the Foundation's Fighting Back program.

Fighting Back was a national demonstration program that had been designed to find out whether it was possible for local organizations and residents to collaborate effectively to reduce the demand for illegal drugs and alcohol in their communities.

When Fighting Back was announced in early 1989, there had been a big response. More than 330 communities—almost triple the number anticipated—had applied for the program's fifteen planning grants, prompting the federal government, shortly thereafter, to launch a major grant initiative of its own, which it named the Community Partnership Demonstration Grant program. The federal program, loosely modeled on Fighting Back, eventually funded 251 additional community initiatives, including many of those represented at the Washington conference.

That was the good news. The large and unusually rapid influx of federal money meant that many applicants who had not been funded through the Fighting Back program could now apply for government grants to enable them to continue their efforts. As a result, many more communities would be helped.

However, it was clear that those communities would need a lot of help in addition to funding. Mounting a comprehensive local substance abuse initiative of this kind was largely uncharted territory, without a clear road map and with no proven models for community leaders to replicate. The Fighting Back grantees at least had the advantage that The Robert Wood Johnson Foundation had established a well-funded National Program Office at Vanderbilt University to provide them with technical assistance.

But what about the others? While the agency responsible for the federal Community Partnership program would surely do its best, the sheer scale of the program, with hundreds of grantees scattered across the map—from Miami, Florida, all the way to Nome, Alaska—posed a staggering logistical challenge. And there were also communities that hadn't received either federal funding or Fighting Back grants.

There was an additional troubling concern—maintaining substance abuse as a national public policy issue. The Washington conference had featured a number of high-profile national figures, including Jack Kemp, at the time President Bush's secretary of housing and urban development, and William Bennett, who had just the day before stepped down as the nation's drug czar. In speech after speech, Kemp, Bennett, and the other speakers had expressed their enthusiastic support for the kind of leadership these new local coalitions were providing in response to the nation's drug crisis.

On the one hand, of course, such recognition was gratifying to the community leaders assembled in the audience. On the other hand, there was concern that between the lines of these speeches, substance abuse was subtly being redefined as a local rather than a national issue—and hence, a local and not a federal responsibility. The fact that the highly visible Bennett had just announced his resignation, to be replaced by the relatively unknown former Florida governor Bob Martinez, only added to the concern.

Not only would the communities need all kinds of information and training, but there would also have to be a way to keep federal policymakers—as well as state officials—engaged. After all, it was federal and state policies on everything from criminal justice and corrections to financing for prevention and treatment that set the boundaries within which local leaders had to operate. If those policies were not sensitive to the realities on the ground, the communities wouldn't stand a chance.

Hearn and Jellinek began to talk about establishing a national center that could serve both as a resource and as a voice for local substance abuse initiatives. The key would be to find the right person to run it—someone who could work both the community and the policy sides of the street and who did not have a particular professional or ideological ax to grind. After considering a number of possible candidates, the Foundation turned to David Rosenbloom, who had served as the commissioner of health and hospitals for the City of Boston between 1975 and 1983 and was a member of the National Advisory Committee for the Fighting Back program.

In April 1991 The Robert Wood Johnson Foundation awarded a planning grant to the Boston University School of Public Health, where Rosenbloom was based, to develop a blueprint for a national resource center for local substance abuse initiatives. Rosenbloom and his team interviewed more than a hundred people across the country to get a sense of what the needs and priorities were and what resources were available.

There wasn't much. Community leaders told Rosenbloom that they felt isolated and that they didn't have access to current information about what was going on in the field. They were aware of some of the academic research on the effectiveness of various prevention and treatment interventions, but they didn't know how to apply those research findings within their communities. They needed help with everything from leadership and organizational development to strategic planning and fundraising. And, sure enough, they wanted to do whatever they could to improve the poor public policy environment within which they were trying to work.

By midsummer, the plan was ready, and in September the Foundation gave the Boston University School of Public Health a twenty-month grant of nearly $2 million to launch the new national resource center, soon to be given the name Join Together.

With the initial funding for Join Together in place, Rosenbloom quickly began recruiting a diverse staff with expertise in substance abuse research and policy, community mobilization, leadership development, communications, and—in a prescient move—the Internet. In the years to come, Join Together was to pioneer the use of the Internet as a powerful vehicle for informing and connecting the many thousands of local groups and individuals across the country working on substance abuse issues. With more than seven thousand individual visitors a day, Join Together Online is considered one of the field's premier Web sites, providing daily news updates, funding information, key facts and trend data, a search engine that can scan a database of more than twenty-five thousand archived substance abuse studies and reports, and extensive links to other Web sites in the field. Along the way, Join Together also developed Quit-Net, an interactive Web site now in active collaboration with eight state and seven county partners around the country, to help smokers overcome their addiction to tobacco.

In addition to its on-line service, Join Together produced and sent out numerous newsletters, reports, and monthly action kits to its rapidly growing mailing list, helping readers keep abreast of relevant trends and issues and offering guidance on specific actions that local leaders could take to address those issues in their communities. But, as useful as these services were, Join Together was designed to be more than simply a sophisticated information clearinghouse. There was, for example, the Join Together Fellows program, which eventually supported over two hundred local leaders like Chicago's Susan Weed, creating linkages among them so that they could support and learn from one another.

Approximately thirty fellows were selected each year for the one-year fellowship. During that year, those fellows would be brought together three times, for four or five days at a time, for intensive sessions on leadership development, strategic planning, and a variety of relevant content areas, such as recent advances in prevention research and updates on new public policy developments in the field. In addition, the meetings allowed ample time for the fellows to get to know one another and to share experiences from their respective communities. Beyond these three core meetings, fellows were invited to special meetings on particular issues or topics relevant to their communities, and were often called upon to make presentations, to meet with policymakers in Washington and elsewhere, and to participate in Join Together's technical assistance site visits to communities. Roberta Garson Leis, Join Together's program director, says of the fellows, "We wove them into everything we do."

To help them stay connected with Join Together and with one another beyond their one-year fellowships, Join Together developed a newsletter and an on-line listserv specifically for the fellows. Over time, Join Together hoped to build a nationwide network of trained, connected individuals who could provide continued leadership in helping to mobilize their communities against substance abuse.

There was also an ambitious hands-on technical assistance program, including a series of "Community Exchanges" through which community leaders could visit and learn from other communities face-to-face. These Community Exchange visits generally included both public forums and private meetings designed to share ideas and to promote broader participation in local efforts to address substance abuse.

Leis recalls a Community Exchange visit she made to Amherst, New York, a middle-class suburb of Buffalo. She brought with her a team of leaders from other communities who had dealt with some of the same issues facing Amherst. During the visit, the team met privately with local clergy, judges, and business leaders; and during the subsequent public forums, one of the clergy and one of the judges openly confronted the parents in the audience about their denial that substance abuse was, in fact, a real problem among Amherst's young people. Following up six months after the Community Exchange, Leis learned that Amherst had enacted new policies addressing underage drinking, that a drug court was being established, and that the number of business leaders in Amherst's substance abuse coalition had increased from three to thirty-five.

Also, to address the concerns that communities might be left in the lurch as the federal government began backing away from the substance abuse issue, Join Together launched a series of public policy panels, modeled after a Twentieth Century Fund (now The Century Fund) panel on which Rosenbloom himself had once served. These panels, which were chaired by prominent public figures and made up of experts and community leaders, developed recommendations that were widely disseminated to public officials and advocates. In an independent survey conducted in the late 1990s, readers of Join Together's many publications ranked the policy panel reports as among the most useful.

Finally, in 1994, Join Together became the National Program Office for the Fighting Back program.

## —w— CADCA

In November 1994, the same month that Susan Weed became Chicago's drug czar, another story was unfolding about two and a half hours southeast of Chicago in Noble County, Indiana. Noble County is a completely different place from Chicago in almost every respect imaginable. "Noble County is the heart of the Northeastern Indian lake area, and is composed of scenic rolling farmland and scattered lakes," says one of the Web sites describing the community. With only about forty-seven thousand residents in the entire county—94 percent of them white—Noble County has fewer people than some city blocks in Chicago.

Yet, like Chicago, Noble County faced a very real substance abuse problem. One of the first community leaders to spot the problem was Judge Michael Kramer of the Noble Superior Court. "I was becoming more and more frustrated seeing the same people coming through the courts—sometimes whole families—and a lot of it because of drugs and alcohol," he recalls. "The fact is that we had nothing going on in the county as far youth goes, and so the predominant culture was drug use, especially among the young people. And it got worse, because it turned out we were on a major drug route."

Kramer had started attending meetings of the local substance abuse coalition, which at that point had only four or five members and some very modest funding provided through local court revenues. "As I became more frustrated, I became very outspoken at our coalition meetings," he says. "I felt we should be doing more. And so in November they elected me chair of the group. Unfortunately, at that time I didn't really know anything about coalitions."

Eventually, like Susan Weed, Kramer learned about Join Together, and today he is one of more than twenty-one thousand subscribers to JTO-Direct, an e-mail service from Join Together Online. But Join Together was not where Kramer first turned for help.

"When I agreed to chair our local coalition, I wanted to see it succeed, but I didn't know what to do," Kramer recalls. "And then, out of the blue, I got a brochure in the mail about a big leadership forum in Washington, D.C., specifically for antidrug coalitions. It was very last minute, but I went anyhow. And when I got there, I just couldn't believe it. It was astounding to see what all these groups were doing all over the country. I went to every workshop I could and listened hard to what they had to say. I learned so much."

As Kramer discovered when he got there, the forum had been convened by another new national organization, also supported by The Robert Wood Johnson Foundation, called "Community Anti-Drug Coalitions of America"—or, as it is generally referred to in the field, "CADCA." It had been launched in October 1992, about a year after Join Together, and for much the same reason: to reduce the isolation of local substance abuse initiatives.

In many ways, CADCA was the brainchild of Alvah Chapman, the former chair and chief executive officer of the Knight Ridder newspaper chain. Chapman was a founder of the Miami Coalition, a group of business and civic leaders who had come together in response to Miami's drug crisis in the late 1980s. In 1989, he had joined the President's Drug Advisory Council.

Because of his involvement with the Miami Coalition, Chapman was asked to chair the council's committee on community coalitions. Shortly after becoming chair, he invited leaders from a dozen local coalitions to meet with his committee in Washington. They all said that they were working in splendid isolation. "There was a common thread to what they said, and that was the need to come together on a regular basis," Chapman recalls. "Getting them together was the best thing we could do."

The upshot was the November 1990 Washington conference. But clearly one conference was not enough. Chapman was keenly aware that the local leaders he had talked with wanted to get together at least once a year. Moreover, with new coalitions springing up every day and the field itself in rapid evolution, there had to be a way to continue to convene the coalitions in the years to come. But who could do it?

The President's Drug Advisory Council was slated to go out of existence in the near future, so that was not an option. The federal government might have done it, but there was a feeling that it would be better to have an independent organization that could not only convene the coalitions but also begin to represent their interests as a group. Join Together, which at that time was still in its formative stage, might have been an option, but Chapman and others on the President's Drug Advisory Council felt strongly that an organization representing the coalitions should be based in or near the nation's capital, not in Boston.

And so the decision was made to start from scratch with a brand-new organization: CADCA. Not only was CADCA to be independent, it was also to be established as a membership organization so that it could legitimately claim to represent the interests of its member coalitions. CADCA set up shop in Alexandria, Virginia, just across the river from Washington, and Chapman became the first chair of its board.

As a member of the board of the John S. and James L. Knight Foundation, Chapman was able to secure a grant from Knight, but more was needed. So the decision was made to approach The Robert Wood Johnson Foundation, which by that time was the largest philanthropic funder in the substance abuse arena. In October 1992, CADCA received an initial two-and-a-half-year grant of $500,000 from The Robert Wood Johnson Foundation to "help establish an organizational base for the several hundred anti-drug community coalitions formed through the efforts of

The Robert Wood Johnson Foundation, the federal Office of Substance Abuse Prevention, and the President's Drug Advisory Council."

The following month, with the ink barely dry on the legal paperwork that formally established it as a tax-exempt charitable organization, CADCA held its first annual National Leadership Forum. Initially, it was touch-and-go. Chapman recalls that two weeks before the meeting, only seventy people had registered. But at the last minute, they were overwhelmed: more than six hundred people showed up. CADCA's National Leadership Forums have proved to be popular ever since. Attendance has steadily increased over the years, surging to a record 1,800 participants for the 2003 meeting.

Not everyone, however, has been a satisfied customer. Susan Weed, for example, brought a group from Chicago to a CADCA Forum in the mid-1990s and recalls that their reaction was "completely negative." She explains, "Our organizations were urban, mostly black and Latino. The presentations just didn't speak to them. So that was the end of our connection with CADCA."

Beverly Watts Davis, formerly the executive director of San Antonio's Fighting Back program and, since May 2003, the director of the federal government's Center for Substance Abuse Prevention, agrees that in its early years CADCA "did not truly reflect the face of America." But in her view there have been dramatic improvements, especially since Arthur Dean, a retired army major general, became CADCA's chair and chief executive officer in 1998. "He has turned the entire situation around," Davis says. "This year [2003] when I went to the conference, I was amazed at the diversity."

An independent survey of several hundred CADCA members and observers conducted in 2000 seems to support Davis's view. In the dry language of the report, "Respondents believe that CADCA maintains an appropriate balance between . . . needs of urban versus suburban and rural areas."

From the outset, despite the obvious importance of its National Leadership Forums, CADCA saw itself as more than simply a convener of coalitions. Like Join Together, CADCA developed an array of services—including training and technical assistance, marketing and communications support, funding information, research updates, legislative alerts, and public policy support—that it believed would strengthen local coalitions. And groups like Kramer's fledgling coalition in Noble County soon began turning to CADCA for help.

"As I listened to what they had to say, it was really almost like a recipe," the judge says, recalling his first CADCA Forum in 1994. "It was a step-by-step process that CADCA helped us to get going on. And when I got back to Noble County, we took what little money we had and sent a teacher with twenty students to a PRIDE [Parents' Resource Institute for Drug Education] conference to do something about the drug culture in the schools. Today we've got about seven hundred students in the schools directly involved, mostly doing community service."

But that was only a first step. With CADCA's help and encouragement, Kramer was eventually able to bring new resources into the community, enabling the coalition to take a more comprehensive approach to reducing demand. "In 1998, we got funded by the federal government's Drug-Free Communities Program, which made it possible for us to get our first paid staff person—and CADCA helped us with that," he explained. "It helped us stabilize the PRIDE program, and now we're also working on treatment. For instance, one problem I had as a judge was the lack of halfway houses. At one point, there was a six-month wait. We now have three halfway houses in the area, and there's no wait anymore. We also helped to start a sliding scale outpatient drug treatment program at the mental health center, and that has helped a lot." He paused. "Don't get me wrong. We still have our problems. For instance, our treatment providers fight a lot."

Over the past decade, Noble County's coalition has gradually grown from the four or five individuals who used to get together over lunch when Kramer first became involved to more than ninety groups and individuals today, including school superintendents, teachers, counselors, large groups of youth, treatment agencies, recovery houses, mental health service providers, judges, probation officers, the county sheriff, local police, state police, parents, people from the local hospital, the county health department, a nurse, clergy, journalists, and the publisher of the local newspaper. Kramer is especially proud of the degree of youth involvement, noting that a high school senior chairs the coalition's prevention committee.

In contrast to the kind of intensive, on-site technical assistance that Amherst, New York, received through Join Together's Community Exchange program, CADCA staff did not come to Noble County to provide technical assistance. Instead, in addition to the National Leadership Forum in Washington, Kramer and his colleagues attended several regional CADCA workshops and training sessions, including a two-day workshop in Indianapolis. Also, there was a great deal of what the judge describes as "informal contact with all the people at CADCA," including frequent telephone calls to "ask for advice and bounce ideas off them."

CADCA's publications were also helpful, especially *Strategizer,* a monthly technical assistance report organized around hot topics in the field that presents various approaches to coalition building, and *Practical Theorist,* a series of reports sponsored by the National Institute on Drug Abuse that summarizes the latest findings from scientific research.

While Kramer and his fellow coalition members appreciate CADCA's guidance and support, in the beginning one of CADCA's most important contributions probably wasn't even visible to most members of Noble County's coalition. And that was CADCA's successful advocacy on Capitol Hill to promote federal funding for substance abuse coalitions—including the Drug-Free Communities Act that provided Noble County's pivotal federal grant in 1998.

Sue Thau, a consultant to CADCA paid solely from membership dues, is widely credited with almost single-handedly leveraging over a billion dollars in federal support for local substance abuse initiatives and for substance abuse prevention, treatment, and research. Before her work in the substance abuse field, Thau spent fifteen years working on appropriations issues at the Office of Management and Budget. According to an independent assessment of CADCA conducted for The Robert Wood Johnson Foundation by Patrizi Associates, "Without question, no other aspect of CADCA's work is more highly regarded than Thau's advocacy activities."

## —✺— Not a Natural Act

At a 2003 meeting of grantees funded under the Fighting Back program, Beverly Watts Davis, the former executive director of the Fighting Back initiative in San Antonio, commented that collaboration—whether to fight a community's substance abuse problem or any of the many other complex health and social challenges currently confronting local leaders—is "not a natural act." That is because true collaboration requires people representing different constituencies and organizations to set aside some of their own immediate factional or institutional self-interests—as well as any historical tensions—in order to achieve a greater common good. Usually, when collaboration does occur, it is short-term, and it is triggered by an especially urgent crisis that affects all parties—a flood, an earthquake, a terrorist attack.

But forging and sustaining collaboration for the long haul in response to a complex, deeply rooted problem such as substance abuse is, as Davis put it, "a very different kettle of fish." It is extraordinarily difficult, often demoralizing work on a problem that many in the community may not even be willing to acknowledge, much less do anything about, and progress can be painfully slow and hard to measure.

Recognizing this, since 1991 The Robert Wood Johnson Foundation has invested more than $45 million in Join Together ($33.6 million) and CADCA ($12.3 million) to support, inform, and connect what have now grown to be thousands of local substance abuse initiatives and coalitions nationwide.

From the outset, this has been a hugely ambitious undertaking for both organizations. It is no surprise, therefore, that just as Chicago's Susan Weed and Noble County's Michael Kramer often found themselves in uncharted territory as they worked to mobilize their communities against substance abuse, so, too, Join Together and CADCA have been on a continual learning curve as they have tried to determine how best to support those thousands of local leaders and coalitions on the front lines. Their task has been complicated by the inherently fluid, and often messy, nature of local collaboration and by the fact that substance abuse remains such a highly charged, stigmatized, and underfunded field.

Despite these complications, both organizations have learned and matured over time, and their experiences in managing some of the issues they encountered during their first dozen years of operation may be instructive to others seeking to support local activity directed at tough health and social problems.

### *Staying on Mission*

Among the most vexing issues that emerged for both Join Together and CADCA during the 1990s was the question of how to remain focused in the face of so many demands from so many different directions. CADCA vice president Mary Elizabeth Larson recalls that when she started working for CADCA in 1997, "We were a fly-by-the-seat-of-your-pants, don't-say-no-to-anybody kind of organization. It was 'love all, serve all.' Unfortunately, when you do that, it takes you off your mission."

This was the issue that faced Arthur Dean when he took the helm as CADCA's chair and chief executive officer in 1998. One of the most important things Dean feels that he has done is to make sure that CADCA stays focused on its primary mission of creating and strengthening the capacity of community coalitions to create safe, healthy, and drug-free communities. This emphasis on strengthening capacity means that, for CADCA, quality has become more important than quantity—or, as Dean puts it, "While growing the coalition field is very important, what is even more important is increasing the effectiveness of each coalition."

In another important respect, however, CADCA has broadened its focus. In contrast to Join Together, which from the outset defined substance abuse broadly and dealt with treatment as well as prevention, CADCA had initially limited its focus to illegal drug abuse and to prevention. "But," says Dean, "when I traveled to coalitions around the country, I became aware of the need to expand our focus to the total demand reduction effort—including treatment, and including alcohol and tobacco." He quickly adds, "Of course, we have kept the focus on *underage* drinking, which is illegal."

Dean's decision to expand CADCA's focus to "the total demand reduction effort" after visiting member coalitions points up a delicate balance that CADCA, as a membership organization, now tries to maintain between "staying on mission" on the one hand while on the other hand staying keenly attuned to the needs and concerns on the front line. Not only does Dean personally continue to spend a good deal of time on the road visiting coalitions, but he has also established a formal advisory committee of a dozen seasoned coalition leaders who meet with CADCA staff every six months to provide input and feedback from the field. And, in what he sees as an especially important move, Dean has appointed a well-respected coalition leader to the position of vice chair for coalition affairs on CADCA's largely corporate board: "to make sure we hear from the coalitions, that we listen to them, and that we look like them."

Like CADCA, Join Together struggled to stay focused during the 1990s. Lack of focus was, in fact, a major theme in an independent assessment of Join Together conducted by Patrizi Associates for The Robert Wood Johnson Foundation in 2000. The report stated, "Join Together is spread too thin," and went on to suggest that Join Together consider taking on the issue of substance abuse treatment as a primary focus.

As it turned out, Join Together director David Rosenbloom had been thinking along the same lines. In 1998, Rosenbloom had approached The Robert Wood Johnson Foundation with the idea of having Join Together do something to expand treatment. Rosenbloom said that he had initially envisioned Join Together simply as a resource center that was there to be responsive to the needs of people in the field. But, as it turned out, people's needs were all over the map. And his work with the Fighting Back communities had convinced him of the importance of doing something about treatment.

Inevitably, the decision to sharpen its focus on treatment forced Join Together to make some difficult trade-offs. For example, as the centerpiece of its enhanced commitment to treatment, Join Together launched a new initiative, named Demand Treatment!, which provided training and technical assistance, together with grants of $60,000, to try to catalyze treatment expansion in twenty-nine cities around the country. At the same time, it phased out the popular Join Together Fellows program, which had been such a boon to Susan Weed and many other community leaders.

A second, obvious trade-off was that more attention to treatment meant less attention to prevention. "While I don't believe that our taking a position on treatment has affected our objectivity and our credibility, it has focused our attention," he says. "And as a result, we are probably spending less time on pure prevention issues. Of course, not everybody is happy about that."

In a sense, Join Together and CADCA have converged on a kind of middle ground in terms of their areas of focus: although CADCA has become far more disciplined about staying on mission, it has broadened its focus to include treatment as well as prevention within its purview, while Join Together, although not abandoning prevention, has narrowed its focus somewhat in order to actively promote treatment. Both Dean and Rosenbloom made these decisions based, at least in part, on what they saw and heard on the front lines—Dean in his visits to member coalitions, Rosenbloom in working with the Fighting Back grantees. The fact that both organizations seem to have picked up similar signals from the field suggests that they are now probably more or less on track.

### Meeting the Demand for Technical Assistance

Along with the challenge of staying focused, the second major issue that both CADCA and Join Together ran into almost immediately was how to keep up with the nearly overwhelming demand for technical assistance. Not that it should have come as a surprise.

It wasn't until their technical assistance staffs got out into the field and started working with real, live communities, however, that the immensity of the challenge became clear. As the report of Patrizi Associates notes, "The sheer issue of scale—that is, delivering sufficient services to a large enough number of coalitions in appropriate magnitude that would allow one to see observable changes in the community—is daunting." In its earlier years, CADCA's technical assistance teams were on the road almost every week of the year, leading to burnout of the technical assistance staff and CADCA's withdrawing from the field.

Things were not much better, if at all, at Join Together. Like CADCA, Join Together in its early years tried the hands-on retail approach to technical assistance, including the popular Community Exchange visits—like the one Roberta Garson Leis and her team conducted in Amherst, New York—in which local leaders visited one another's communities to share experiences and insights.

But Rosenbloom and his staff, too, soon discovered that such an approach was far too labor intensive for a market as big as Join Together's and that new methods would have to be found—if not to replace the site visits, then certainly to supplement them. While CADCA, with its constituency limited to community coalitions, today has just over five thousand dues-paying and associate members, Join Together's master mailing list of local officials, agencies, organizations, and coalitions of all shapes and sizes currently includes upward of eighty thousand names.

Enter the Internet. From the beginning, when he was working on the initial blueprint for Join Together, Rosenbloom had become fascinated by the potential of this new communications technology. But he kept his aspirations modest initially. "When we started, nobody knew what we were talking about," he says. "Our original goal was that at the end of the first five years, eight hundred people would use our electronic information." Today, twelve years later, Join Together has twenty-one thousand subscribers to its electronic newsletter alone, and more than seven thousand people visit Join Together's Web site each day. In addition, content from Join Together Online is syndicated to approximately three hundred other Web sites (including CADCA's), greatly expanding its reach.

What has made this seismic shift possible is not just improvements in the technology but also what Rosenbloom describes as a fundamental change in user attitudes and behavior. "In the beginning, we literally had to pay people's fees for them to use this stuff," he says. "Now people have become more self-sufficient and self-directed. So technical assistance that in the beginning required several full-time staff members and only helped a few people a day is now largely self-directed by people's ability to search our Web site and others. Our Web site is constructed so that every time someone gets information from it, links to other information on the same topic appear. All of this means that we can help thousands of people a day instead of just a few."

Despite the huge surge in its delivery of on-line technical assistance, Join Together has not cut back its traditional hands-on technical assistance capacity. "We still have five staff people who do site visits and use the telephone and e-mail and snail mail, and we still get about a hundred requests a month, the same as before. We tried to phase it out, but they just kept calling," Rosenbloom says wistfully.

In contrast, CADCA did phase out its hands-on technical assistance operation in the mid-1990s, largely as a result of staff burnout. However, shortly after Dean's arrival in 1998, CADCA made an abrupt about-face and rebuilt its technical assistance capability. Convinced that technical assistance was vital to CADCA's mission of strengthening the capacity of coalitions, Dean brought on new staff members and charged them with developing new ways of getting help to those who needed it.

As a result, CADCA, in partnership with the National Guard, began using distance learning technology to deliver technical assistance through more than three thousand satellite downlink sites around the country. CADCA also significantly upgraded its Web site as a vehicle for technical assistance, although, as Dean notes, "We don't rival Join Together Online because we focus on serving our members, not the field as a whole."

In addition, CADCA began making greater use of sessions and workshops at its National Leadership Forum as technical assistance opportunities. And finally, recognizing—as Join Together did—that there were continuing requests for hands-on aid, CADCA restored at least some of its capacity to provide technical assistance by telephone and on-site, albeit with a less grueling site visit regimen than in the past.

These changes, however, were only a first step. In September 2002, CADCA was awarded a $2 million federal grant—its first ever—to establish a new National Community Anti-Drug Coalition Institute. Making use of trained mentors, state and regional training sessions, partnerships with key federal agencies, and a panel of scientific advisers, the institute focuses its efforts on improving the way coalitions use data for strategic planning purposes, strengthening their leadership and operations, supporting their use of sound coalition principles and evidence-based interventions, and enhancing their ability to track the impact they are having.

How the new institute will pan out remains to be seen. There is no question, however, that both CADCA and Join Together have already taken major steps during their first decade of operations to revamp their initial retail approach to technical assistance. Although there are obvious differences in some of the specific elements of their technical assistance programs, both organizations have pursued the same basic strategy of moving to more of a wholesale approach, and both have capitalized on technological advances such as the Internet and satellite communications to help them do so.

Yet, at the same time, neither organization has so far felt comfortable completely abandoning the traditional hands-on approach. Not only is there still a demand in the field for the human touch, but—as the leaders of both organizations have themselves discovered—being out in the field remains an indispensable way for any organization to keep its ear to the ground.

### Advancing Public Policy

CADCA and Join Together have been active on the public policy front almost from the beginning. Both organizations have consistently viewed public policy as a critically important dimension of their work. However, there was—and to a large extent there still is—a fundamental difference in their focus and their approach. CADCA's primary public policy emphasis has been on *funding*—with particular attention to federal funding for local antidrug coalitions—while Join Together's emphasis has been on a wide range of *contextual* policy issues that community leaders have identified as especially relevant to their local substance abuse efforts, such as underage drinking statutes and criminal justice policies.

Although there is some overlap in practice, the basic difference in emphasis is likely to persist. As a membership organization, CADCA can legitimately speak for the interests of its members, including their financial interests. On issues like underage drinking and criminal justice, on the other hand, Join Together's status as an objective, university-based resource center that does *not* officially represent any particular constituency gives it a kind of credibility that a membership organization generally does not have.

At one point in the mid-1990s, there was some discussion at The Robert Wood Johnson Foundation about encouraging Join Together and CADCA to merge into a single organization, primarily for reasons of economic efficiency. One of the principal reasons the Foundation ultimately decided not to go down that road was the recognition that both organizations played important roles in the substance abuse policy arena, but they were roles that could not be combined within a single organization.

### Building the Substance Abuse Field

Finally, a pervasive and inescapable issue that both Join Together and CADCA have faced from day one—the proverbial elephant in the middle of the room—has been the state of the substance abuse field itself.

When talking about CADCA's constituents, Dean makes the point that "these communities are working on America's number one health problem." But it is a problem that many Americans are unwilling to acknowledge, either within their own lives or within their communities, largely because of the profound social stigma that is still associated with substance abuse. This same stigma affects many of those who choose to work in the substance abuse field, in terms of both professional status and earnings—a fact that has kept many of the best and the brightest from considering careers in the field. And, to top it off, the field remains bitterly divided at almost every level: supply reduction versus demand reduction; prevention versus treatment; even one form of treatment versus another.

Yet while these realities have clearly made things much more difficult for everyone in the field, including Join Together and CADCA, it may turn out in the long run that one of the most important contributions to emerge from the work of Join Together and CADCA will be the ways in which their various programs and activities have helped to build and strengthen the substance abuse field itself: increasing its funding; enhancing its legitimacy on Capitol Hill; raising its technological sophistication; drawing hundreds of new leaders into the field; strengthening interorganizational linkages; and supporting and encouraging the many thousands of individuals fighting the substance abuse problem in their home communities.

What makes this field-building aspect of their work especially important is the fact that substance abuse—perhaps in contrast to some of the other issues facing local leaders—is such a stubborn, deeply rooted problem. Even when there is progress against one kind of substance abuse, sooner or later another equally dangerous substance crops up, and the battle starts all over again. It is not a field that lends itself to quick and easy solutions, and consequently, whatever can be done to strengthen capacity and leadership for the long haul is likely to yield significant dividends in the years to come.

## —ɯ— The Future

Reflecting on the experiences of Join Together to date, Rosenbloom says, "I believe we've demonstrated that there is a need and a role for this kind of capacity to support what communities are doing. That doesn't mean that we have to be the ones to do it, but the response we've gotten suggests clearly that we're providing services that people want and need."

"However," he adds, "it is also clear that the field is not yet strong enough to support this kind of activity on its own—especially when you still have secretaries who make more money than many of the people who work full-time providing treatment and prevention services."

While CADCA's funding base is considerably more diversified than Join Together's, Dean acknowledges that with only 7 percent of its revenues coming from membership dues (although he hopes to raise it to 12 percent), CADCA, too, will remain dependent on external funders for the foreseeable future.

In other words, while capacity-building organizations like Join Together and CADCA clearly are valued by those they serve, the fact that their constituents do not have sufficient resources to support them on their own means that there can be no guarantees about the future.

Whatever the ultimate future of Join Together and CADCA, the question of how best to support local problem solving and collaboration is likely to resurface with increasing frequency in the years to come as more of the nation's health and social problems are left to communities to resolve for themselves—including everything from the current obesity epidemic to preparedness for a possible bioterrorist attack. Like Susan Weed and Michael Kramer, those community leaders who are on the front lines struggling to cope with these challenges will undoubtedly need ways to get access to information, to navigate the policy shoals, and to support and learn from one another. Perhaps the experiences of CADCA and Join Together can help point the way.

# 3

# The Robert Wood Johnson Foundation's Efforts to Contain Health Care Costs

*Carolyn Newbergh*

---

## Editors' Introduction

Health care now consumes 14 percent of the nation's gross domestic product and is rising at a rate far faster than inflation. This is a matter of concern because high costs make health insurance and, more generally, medical care unaffordable for many, and it leads to an unfair system where those with means have access to excellent care and those without are often forced to do with no or lower-quality care.

This is not a new problem. For many years, the nation has struggled to find ways to contain health care costs and increase access to medical care, as has The Robert Wood Johnson Foundation. In this chapter, Carolyn Newbergh, a freelance writer specializing in health care and a frequent contributor to The Robert Wood Johnson Foundation *Anthology,* examines the logic behind the Foundation's cost containment strategies, discusses how they evolved over the years, and provides an in-depth look at some of the Foundation's major cost containment programs.

Newbergh finds that the Foundation has had an ambivalent attitude toward cost containment. It has gone from a lack of interest in its early years, to declaring cost containment a goal and then lowering it to a half goal, and finally to making it simply a component of most of its health care programs. Nonetheless, the Foundation has devoted substantial resources to cost containment—in excess of $250 million over the past twenty-two years. And this is really an underestimate, since cost containment is an implicit element in programs designed to increase coverage and to better understand the health care system and how it is financed.

The Foundation's ambivalence toward cost containment is largely the result of uncertainty about the ability of a foundation—even one the size of Robert Wood Johnson—to affect the course of a $1.4 trillion industry. Whether foundations should nibble on the margins of large social problems (where they are more likely to have a small but measurable impact) or whether they should launch a full assault (where the chances for failure are greater) is an issue that should engage not just The Robert Wood Johnson Foundation but philanthropy as a whole.

A s the year 2003 dawned, more than two dozen orthopedic, heart, and general surgeons walked off the job at four West Virginia hospitals to protest sky-high malpractice premiums, leaving in the lurch patients who might need emergency surgery. One doctor said that in his twenty-two years in practice, his premium had shot up from $800 to $160,000 annually. "Our group can't do business," he said. "We're broke." Restive surgeons in other states threatened their own demonstrations.

A week later came another sign that the American health care system wasn't well. The government came out with statistics showing that health care spending was at its highest level ever, making up 14.1 percent of the nation's gross domestic product, or GDP. The *New York Times* reported that "spending on health care is increasing at the fastest rate in a decade."

Over the past twenty-five years, the American public has been regularly subjected to news bulletins like these that scream out about a health care crisis du jour. Ambulances turned away from overcrowded emergency rooms. Seniors going without food so they can buy the expensive prescription drugs they need. Managed care horror stories of treatments denied. Double-digit increases in insurance premiums. An unconscionable number of uninsured people that continues to mushroom. Health care costs rising faster than GDP—grabbing too much of consumers' hard-earned income and threatening the ability of American business to remain competitive globally.

And over and over, during the crises in the health care system that peaked in the early 1980s, 1990s, and the past few years—coinciding with national economic downturns—there has been sufficient blame to go around. Some point their fingers at greedy hospitals, doctors, pharmaceutical companies, and insurers. Others say the biggest culprit is overuse of the medical system by patients—often elderly ones—who have insatiable appetites for costly diagnostic tests and the latest that technology can do for them or who live unhealthy lifestyles. Still others zero in on the way the health care system is financed, offering too many incentives for doctors and hospitals to spend wastefully and function inefficiently.

Numerous antidotes have been prescribed over the years, with various degrees of success—including price controls; certificate-of-need programs to limit hospital beds and redundant technology; utilization review to prevent unnecessary care; malpractice reform; Medicare's prospective payment system to lower reimbursements for hospitals and doctors; Medicaid's cutbacks in eligibility and benefits; managed care with its capitation and gatekeepers; pushing operations out of hospitals and into outpatient surgery centers; medical practice guidelines for particular health problems; and higher deductibles and copayments that transfer some of the cost burden to patients.

"We have a cycle of blame shifting, cost shifting, and causal analysis shifting," said Lawrence Brown, a Columbia University public health professor. "When you try to think about strategies to address the cost issue, it gets fragmented awfully fast—there are so many causal elements and places you could focus your resources and attention on."

There have been brief periods when health care cost inflation seems to have been tamed, particularly in managed care's heyday in the mid- to late 1990s. Yet runaway health costs persist. Fixing one piece of the puzzle seems to simply pawn the cost off elsewhere in the system in an elaborate cost-shifting game.

"The problem as I see it is that it's been like squeezing balloons," said Steven Schroeder, former Robert Wood Johnson Foundation president and chief executive officer. "Fundamentally, you have surges in demand and supply. You can put the brakes on by changing how you reimburse, being more efficient, moving care out of the hospital, lowering malpractice costs, and lowering the tendency to do defensive medicine. All of those kinds of things would be helpful. If you do them all at once, you might have a perfect storm for cost containment, but it's really hard to do them all at once."

## —◊— The Robert Wood Johnson Foundation's Approaches to Cost Containment: 1972–2003

Throughout these tumultuous times for the health care industry, The Robert Wood Johnson Foundation has struggled to define what role it should play in cost containment. In its fledgling days in the early 1970s, the Foundation stayed out of the cost debate, pursuing its goals of improving access to and quality of care. Because many staff members and trustees believed that national health insurance was right around the corner, the Foundation looked for ways to help expand the health care system's capacity to meet the anticipated increased demand. This led the Foundation to focus its efforts in areas such as helping to develop hospital group practices, nurse practitioners and physician assistants, the emergency medical services system, community health centers, and regional perinatal care networks. The Foundation addressed cost issues only indirectly. If, for example, it turned out that using nurse practitioners to extend quality care to more people also happened to lower health care costs, that was a nice by-product, but not the intended purpose of the nurse practitioner program.

As health care costs climbed later in the 1970s, however, sitting on the sidelines became increasingly uncomfortable for the Foundation. "A lot of distinguished people were very critical of us over the years because high costs were driving everyone crazy," said Robert Blendon, a former senior vice president, who helped lead the Foundation from its inception in 1972 to 1986. "But both the board of trustees and David Rogers [the Foundation's first president] always felt that their passion was not saving money but giving better care to people who couldn't get it. Their thinking was that government and business should worry about saving money."

A turning point came when costs spiraled further skyward in the early 1980s, rising faster than the overall economy, which was sputtering into deep recession. Those who led the Foundation felt that the time had come when the nation's largest health care philanthropy had to become part of the solution. In his 1980 president's statement in the Foundation's *Annual Report*, Rogers noted just how pressing health care cost inflation had become. "The public now lists high costs as the single most important problem facing American medicine, and when polled independently, physicians agree," he wrote. He worried that some of the remarkable gains of the 1970s in access to care for the poor, which the Foundation and others had fought for, would be lost as economic resources shrank.

Rogers went on to state that the Foundation was stepping out in a new direction by including cost as one of its three goals (the other two were improving access for the underserved and helping the ill and the disabled to function as highly as possible). Under the new goal, the Foundation would support programs "to make health care arrangements more effective and care more affordable." The idea was to fund research, development, and demonstration projects aimed at slowing the rate at which health care costs rise while still maintaining the quality of care.

In 1982, Rogers announced what would be the Foundation's largest effort in the 1980s focused exclusively on containing costs, Community Programs for Affordable Health Care. This effort sprang from the many notions percolating up around the country on how to rein in runaway health care costs at the local level, particularly an idea in Rochester, New York, that had been successful in marshaling community leaders to hold costs down. Community Programs for Affordable Health Care would use a community coalition model in the hope that major interest groups— business, labor, physicians, hospitals, and insurers—sitting around a table would find bold, imaginative ways to lower costs for the common good. This voluntary approach could then be reproduced in other communities.

The Foundation also kicked off a number of other cost-related initiatives in the early and mid-1980s: the Physician-Directed Program to Improve Medical Care Services and Control Costs, the Program for Prepaid Managed Health Care, the Faculty Fellowships in Health Care Financing, and the Program for Research and Development on Health Care Costs, which would evolve over the years into today's Changes in Health Care Financing and Organization.

In 1987, Leighton Cluff, who was then president of the Foundation, included the organization and financing of health services among the Foundation's ten new "areas of particular concern." He noted that there had been "sweeping changes" in how the medical care system was organized and that financing methods had "undergone something of a revolution over the past twenty years." The Foundation would fund grants that looked at the "systematic reorganization" of how health care was delivered and paid for and would also support health care policy analysis.

By 1990, the Foundation had authorized an estimated $192 million for a patchwork of grants related to cost containment, financing, and related issues. Reflecting the evolving understanding of this field, there was disagreement about what actually constituted cost containment efforts and whether grants aimed at health care financing and related issues were in fact true cost containment measures. But nearly everyone at the Foundation did agree on one thing—that none of the programs had produced the kind of impact in holding down health care costs that had been hoped for.

Schroeder stepped into his new post as Foundation president in 1990 with a definite predilection. His own scholarly research into the financial incentives doctors have to overuse expensive technologies had shown him the limited ability of studies to bring about lower costs in the health care system—even when the research draws much attention, as his did.

"When I got here, there was some pressure from the board to take costs on in a bigger way," Schroeder said. "I didn't want to do it. I knew quite a bit about this field. It seemed to me that the drivers of medical costs were the diffusion of technology, patient demand, the way care is reimbursed, the policies of insurance companies—and those were all outside of what we could do much about. The Foundation just didn't have any leverage to use."

In his first presidential message, in 1990, Schroeder named three goals and subordinated cost to what later became a "half goal." Nevertheless, Schroeder said at the time that the Foundation would "seek opportunities to help the nation address, effectively and fairly, the overarching problem of escalating medical care expenditures." He cited the inability of numerous efforts within the Foundation and without to wrestle down cost inflation. "Since there is little likelihood that we or anyone else will forge a 'magic bullet' to solve the problem of cost, our efforts will embrace a system-wide approach, involving many separate interventions. These will include support for policy analysis to inform the cost containment debate, exercise of our convening powers to bring appropriate leaders together, and health services research."

Meanwhile, some Foundation staff members felt that by downgrading cost containment to half goal status, such issues as affordability and health care financing would get short shrift. They also worried that this might be the first step toward folding cost into other goals, thus reducing their ability to look broadly at what was going on in the health care market.

"We may not have been able to do much about cost containment per se, but there were many of us who felt we needed to learn a lot more and could have an impact on influencing health care financing," said Nancy Barrand, a senior program officer.

During the early 1990s, the Foundation concentrated its efforts on costs in a special staff work group that oversaw grants for analytical work and demonstration projects in health care financing and the Changes in Health Care Financing and Organization, or HCFO, program, which funded research, demonstrations, and evaluations on the financing of health care delivery systems. By the mid-1990s, when managed care brought growth in health care spending under control for several years, the Foundation established its ambitious Health Tracking initiative to monitor this new marketplace approach and any possible fallout.

As it turned out, cost containment lasted as a half goal for five years, and then in 1996 was blended into the Foundation's other goals. The 1996 *Annual Report* noted that "controlling costs is clearly an essential prerequisite for our other goals of assuring access to care, improving services for people with chronic illnesses, and expanding efforts to prevent and treat the harm caused by substance abuse."[1] In 1998, cost containment was added to the Foundation's access goal: "To assure that all Americans have access to basic health care at reasonable cost."[2]

In hindsight, one can see that the story of how the Foundation's role in health care costs evolved in the 1990s is really that of how a strong leader with a clear vision of what is and isn't possible for an organization holds his troops to that vision. "We haven't done cost containment because I sort of threw cold water on it when it came up," Schroeder said. "Not that I didn't think the cost issue was critical. I think it is very important. But I didn't see what advantage this Foundation had."

Over time, the cost half goal simply petered out, he said. "Gradually, the half a goal atrophied to a quarter of a goal, and then finally we went to the board and said, 'We're not really able to sustain this as a goal anymore, so let's quietly bury it,'" he said. "It was a nonevent. It was a very quiet interment without 'Taps' or flowers."

Through 2003, the Foundation had spent somewhere between $250 million and $500 million in grants that in some way touched on cost. The wide range stems from uncertainty about what to consider as a cost containment grant. When staff members were asked which grants aimed at cost over all these years stand out as having made a difference or having pointed the way, there was near unanimous head scratching. No shining examples sprang to mind. And there was little agreement among staff members about cost containment programs that were at least worthwhile or highly interesting. Their choices seem to reflect their own personal interests, indicating that cost containment is in the eye of the beholder. These are some highlights:

- Schroeder praised the Foundation's support since the early 1990s of the *Dartmouth Atlas of Health Care in the United States,* a regularly updated book by John Wennberg of the Dartmouth Medical School showing that health care spending is much higher in some regions of the country with greater supplies of hospitals and doctors but with no resulting benefit in health outcomes. In other words, more health care is not necessarily better health care. Wennberg has been an advocate of improving health care access without more spending by cutting back in areas in which too much care is given. His work has had enormous influence on the thinking about what is necessary care or too much care.

- Some mentioned the On Lok approach to care for the elderly, an HMO model in which one provider managed all the acute and long-term care for the frail elderly. This program succeeded in its main goal, to bring high-quality care to the elderly in a managed care setting, but secondarily also reduced costs some. It has been replicated, but not as broadly as had been hoped.

- The studies carried out under the HCFO program on risk adjustment were cited as pioneering and particularly useful. Under a risk adjustment system, an employer pool or health plan pool would pay more to the insurer that enrolled more sick people and less to one that enrolled just the healthiest.

- The Center for Studying Health System Change's regular reports on the cost impact of managed care have become an important and trusted source of information for the public, policymakers, and researchers, others said. The center, in Washington, D.C., is the centerpiece of the Health Tracking initiative and conducts regular surveys to pick up changes in the health care marketplace and understand what they mean. The annual cost reports, produced since 1996 by the center's president, Paul Ginsburg, from data outside the surveys, have been recognized as an early warning system about trends in underlying health services costs and insurance premiums. Also, the many other Foundation grants that examined managed care produced a balanced and needed look at the pros and cons of this health care delivery approach that swept the nation in the 1990s, some said.

- The Foundation has played a vital role in building the capability and capacity of the field of health services research and policy analysis, according to some staff members. Particularly through the highly regarded meetings it sponsors, the Foundation has fostered debate on the major health policy issues of the day relating to costs, financing methods, and health care organization.

Many Foundation staff members have also come to believe that cost implications are inherent in virtually all the Foundation's programs. They point to a wide assortment of programs, including those dealing with health care for the uninsured, increasing access to medical care, improving end-of-life care, medical malpractice, nurse practitioners, workers' compensation, long-term care insurance, care of those with chronic mental illness, and health care reform at the state level. The way this thinking goes, a program to provide better care for people with chronic illnesses, say, will usually turn out to be more affordable, too. "I would say cost is an element in most things we're working on, but it's not the lead element," said Robert Hughes, coordinator of special projects at the Foundation. "It's sort of woven throughout."

Even with a track record of worthy programs to look back on, many current and former Foundation staff members have come to agree with Schroeder that the Foundation cannot have any real impact on a trillion-dollar-plus health care industry. Its place, they say, is not to have a central role in solving the problem of rising health care costs but, from the margins, to advance the knowledge base and stimulate a national conversation on the major cost-related issues. "It's a fantasy for any foundation to believe it can fundamentally influence health care costs in the nation," said Drew Altman, who heads the Henry J. Kaiser Family Foundation in Menlo Park, California, and who stewarded a number of cost containment initiatives while at The Robert Wood Johnson Foundation from 1981 to 1986. "Health care has become dominated by money, Congress, and for-profit medicine, and it's an arena you cannot control. What a foundation can do is produce useful information on health care costs. It can inform the discussion of those who do have leverage. The health care system is now too big and too affected by politics for foundations to have the direct ability to bring about change."

But there are others who believe the Foundation could have done more. Bruce Vladeck, an assistant vice president of the Foundation in 1982 and 1983 who subsequently headed the federal Health Care Financing Administration (now the Centers for Medicare & Medicaid Services), found the Foundation's approach to cost containment lacking. "I disagree with the assessment that the Foundation can't have an impact on costs," he said. "Foundations should be able to say something major about costs and have an impact. I don't know how work on cost containment is different from anything else a foundation does that takes time to show results. You can publish data on beta-blockers reducing the risk of heart attacks, and it takes twenty years for most cardiologists to change their practice patterns, but it does come. The Foundation needed some strategy for advancing a particular set of ideas or proposals or activities, and my sense is they never had such a strategy."

## ⟶ Community Programs for Affordable Health Care

The one major demonstration program mounted by the Foundation directly to contain costs was the Community Programs for Affordable Health Care, or CPAHC. When Ronald Reagan took office in 1980, despite many governmental cost containment efforts attempted in the 1970s, health care spending had reached what was then an all-time high, and the nation was in recession. The rate of growth in hospital spending was increasing at an annual rate of 20 percent in 1980.

Employers were concerned that jumps in health care spending meant that they had to pick up more of the cost of health benefits for their employees, their dependents, and retirees. As a result, business coalitions had begun forming in the late 1970s to negotiate better premium rates with insurers. Another response was coming from communities, which were trying to find ways to clamp a lid on rising costs themselves, before the government or market forces did it for them. Most notable among them was the Rochester, New York, experiment, where nine hospitals, the largest employers, and the two major insurers joined together to restrain the growth in hospital expenses. This leadership group capped the amount that the insurers would pay the local hospitals. It also controlled the hospitals' spending on technology and new service needs by administering a special fund that took the community's overall needs into account. This was the first self-regulated, community-based program to actually hold down hospital spending—and to the slowest rate of spending in the nation.

Many communities interested in a similar strategy approached the Foundation, and vice presidents Robert Blendon and Drew Altman met with top leaders and thinkers of this community coalition concept around the country. Their input helped design CPAHC, a large, multisite national experiment to see if a coalition of community stakeholders— not-for-profit hospitals and insurers, major employers, labor, doctors, and local government—could find creative, groundbreaking ways to restrain rising health costs locally without sacrificing quality or access to care. Although the $17.5 million, seven-year program began operating in 1982, the eleven demonstration sites didn't start up until 1984.

It was an idealistic, sunny notion—and particularly American, many said—that community representatives holding very different vested interests would voluntarily put aside their own needs and aspirations to find a solution to a problem for the greater good. Expectations were high that CPAHC might produce tangible results, such as slowing the rise in expenditures, keeping premiums from their relentless climb, and providing models that could spread to other communities. The Foundation specified that it would be interested in making grants that would support new ways to finance health care (such as changes in incentives and reimbursements to doctors) and to integrate all of a community's local health care services.

It seemed at the start that CPAHC was set up auspiciously. The program was cosponsored by the American Hospital Association and the Blue Cross Blue Shield Association. Its day-to-day operations were headed by Robert Sigmond, a well-regarded leader known for promoting a community leadership model that stressed transcending individual interests to arrive at what is best for the community as a whole. Its National Advisory Committee was led by John Dunlop, a former secretary of labor, who was then an emeritus professor of economics at Harvard University. Dunlop favored community coalitions that arrived at consensus through negotiation. The National Advisory Committee consisted of an elite group including leaders from the American Hospital Association, the Health Insurance Association of America, the American Medical Association, the AFL-CIO, Blue Cross Blue Shield, and the United States Chamber of Commerce.

Even so, there was some skepticism—even within The Robert Wood Johnson Foundation itself—that a cooperative community approach would work. "We had a difference of opinion about whether we could do it," said Blendon, who, with Altman, was a prime mover of the program. "I felt the Foundation had a legitimate role to encourage voluntary groups to see if something could come out of it. I felt it could be productive." For his part, Altman saw that it might be valuable, even noble, to give the private voluntary forces the opportunity to rein in costs themselves. But, he says, "I went into it with the expectation that it couldn't be successful but it was important for the country to try."

The eleven sites selected to participate—Atlanta; Boston; Detroit; Iowa; Mecklenburg County (North Carolina); Minneapolis–St. Paul; New York City; Pittsburgh; Topeka; Tulsa; and Worcester, Massachusetts—had four years to implement their strategies for restraining costs. They tried a number of different approaches: Detroit, for example, emphasized reducing outpatient surgery while Worcester promoted the use of health maintenance organizations.

As time went on, however, the Foundation's leadership came to believe that nothing truly different or innovative was being tested. Instead, many of the projects focused on utilization review of patient services and other approaches that were not brand-new or trailblazing. "They used the lamest strategies in the world," said Alan Cohen, at the time a Foundation vice president who monitored the outside evaluation of CPAHC.

The Foundation's staff became increasingly concerned that the star-studded National Advisory Committee was a major part of the problem. The committee was being run almost as its own private club. And each member had veto power over any project that might be recommended for approval. "I thought this was an embarrassment," said Bruce Vladeck, the former Foundation official. "It was basically saying we're only going to fund something to the extent all the existing power structure supports it, which meant nothing significant would happen."

A blisteringly critical evaluation of CPAHC by Lawrence Brown of Columbia University and Catherine McLaughlin of the University of Michigan confirmed the worst fears. Published in *Health Affairs* in 1990, the Foundation-commissioned evaluation concluded that the program had come up empty-handed, with no models for slowing the rise in health care costs.[3] For many key indicators, such as hospital spending, outpatient surgery, lengths of stay in the hospital, and hospital admission rates, the program sites did no better than the sites with which they were compared. "There is little indication in the data . . . that the rate of growth of health spending in CPAHC sites slowed in contrast with comparable communities outside the program," the evaluators concluded.

Even when sites appeared to show declines in spending, the evaluators said, they could almost always be explained away by looking at trend lines—either at the sites themselves or occurring nationally—that had begun before the program's funding or by the much greater impact of the Medicare system, introduced in 1983, of reimbursing hospital care by diagnostic-related groups.

What had gone so wrong? To the evaluators, it was fairly simple: the program had always been a "mission impossible." Expecting community leaders to exert the discipline needed to slow the growth of health costs without shifting costs or reducing care to the disadvantaged was politically naive; "the program's reach vastly exceeded the communities' grasp," the evaluators wrote. Effective cost containment strategies entail making tough choices, such as paying lower salaries, imposing restrictions, and contracting with certain doctors and not others. But community leaders, who prefer to be known for expanding and improving their community's health care services, didn't want to gore anyone's ox. "Because no one would do anything that affected anyone around the table, they got the lowest-common-denominator projects that had been tried in other places, and nothing audacious," evaluator Lawrence Brown said in an interview. "Not much about cost containment was accomplished. Maybe there were some improvements in local service delivery. No harm done."

Steven Schroeder and coauthors Alan Cohen and Joel Cantor, both then senior officials at The Robert Wood Johnson Foundation, got to the crux of CPAHC's shortcomings in a companion *Health Affairs* article. "The program's central flaw, perhaps, was its misguided assumption that cost containment could be achieved through intervention at the community or local level, when the true levers of power and control existed (and still exist) at the national and state levels of the health care system," the three authors wrote.[4]

In an article in the same issue of *Health Affairs,* John Dunlop, the National Advisory Committee chair, and George Stiles, a CPAHC grantee, vehemently defended the program. The authors charged that Brown and McLaughlin misinterpreted the program's objectives and results and didn't understand the constraints it was under. "Some CPAHC activities produced impressive results in a relatively short time," Dunlop and Stiles wrote. "It is ludicrous to believe, however, that the modest CPAHC resources could demonstrate major community-wide savings (especially in larger cities such as New York and Detroit) in four years or less."[5]

CPAHC did not disprove that community forces can play a part in tackling health costs, they asserted. "Issues involving delivery of services require action at the community level, where the critical clinical decisions that significantly influence cost and quality are made," they wrote. "Problems of physician practice patterns, coordination and integration of services, utilization and managed care, data systems, and so on, need to be addressed at the community level."

Despite the rebuttal by Dunlop and Stiles, the predominant view was that the program had failed.

The evaluators closed their critique with an upbeat silver lining. "Often, in health affairs, understanding what has failed is as important as—and a natural prelude to—discovering what might work." In fact, it seems that

Foundation staff members did make the most of this disappointing enterprise. Although they certainly smarted from the critique's harsh assessment at first, many later said they found it very valuable to have an honest, candid appraisal from which they could gain insight useful to future programming. For example, the Foundation learned where community coalitions can and cannot best be used, and thus has turned to them for such endeavors as the substance abuse and homeless health care programs.

"CPAHC was a disaster for many reasons, but we learned from it," Nancy Barrand, a Foundation senior program officer, said in an interview, echoing the remarks of other staff members. "We learned about the voluntary sector politics and how special interests play out. Even though on paper and in public we're all holding hands as a community coalition, when it comes down to the bottom line business, it's a matter of what is in your self-interest. What are you in business to do if you're an insurance company—save the world? Probably not. What are you in business to do if you're a hospital? Is it to provide free care to everybody? No. We were naive then. Now, as result of CPAHC and some other experiences, we're no longer naive."

## —⁓— Other Programs Related to Cost Containment

The Robert Wood Johnson Foundation has undertaken several initiatives in addition to CPAHC that have included an element of cost control or that were in some way related to cost containment.

### The Physician-Directed Program to Improve Medical Care Services and Control Costs

With fervor to cut health care costs building in the 1980s, many physicians were becoming sensitive to their central role in determining how health care dollars are spent. They were estimated to influence anywhere from 50 to 80 percent of all decisions on health care spending—from when and for how long patients will go to the hospital to whether they will have lab work and X rays. Some approached the Foundation, eager to test ways to put their house in order by themselves rather than have a solution forced on them by the government or private insurers. As a result, the Foundation launched the $2.3 million Physician-Directed Program to Improve Medical Care Services and Control Costs, which ran from 1983 to 1986.

A number of factors had led doctors to err on the side of doing more rather than less—their training to do all they can for a patient's benefit without regard to cost; fear of malpractice lawsuits; and the way fee-for-service health insurance covered all medical expenses, leaving no incentive to cut out wasteful services. The Physician-Directed Program to Improve Medical Care Services and Control Costs provided funds for research and demonstration projects aimed at finding ways for physicians to stop giving patients more medical resources than they needed and to change some of the assumptions about how they practice. The following are some highlights from a sampling of grants that were awarded under the program:

- A Boston University Center for Industry and Health Care utilization management project looked into whether physicians, if given information comparing their own medical practice patterns with others, would reduce their patients' time in the hospital and the testing they ordered for certain common conditions. Although use of services went down a bit at first, the drop did not hold up as this project came to an end. Also, the study could not get all the data it needed to inform the doctors about their practice patterns.

- A three-year University of California, Los Angeles, School of Medicine study created a method for determining the appropriateness of six common medical and surgical procedures, including coronary angiography, coronary artery bypass surgery, and colonoscopy. The investigators said their approach, which they hoped to extend to fifty procedures, held the potential to improve quality while reducing costs.

- A University of Pennsylvania School of Medicine study analyzed the costs and variations in use patterns of sixteen diagnostic services, such as urine cultures, CT scans, ultrasounds, X rays, and electrocardiograms at sixty-three hospitals in five regions. The three-year study found a strong link between the use of these tests and hospital size, number of residents and fellows in relation to beds, and length of patients' stay.

- The Maine Medical Association was given a grant to continue and evaluate a program to encourage Maine doctors to examine variations in surgery rates and, by eliminating unnecessary operations, to reduce costs. This project built on work by one of its coprincipal investigators, John Wennberg. Under the grant, local doctors received feedback on differences in surgery rates and met in small groups to agree on appropriate treatment for certain conditions.

### *The Program for Prepaid Managed Health Care*

The Foundation's $20.4 million Program for Prepaid Managed Health Care, cosponsored with the federal Health Care Financing Administration and the National Governors Association, was a six-year (1984–1990) effort to bring managed care tools, such as case management and capitation, to low-income people receiving Medicaid benefits. A primary care doctor working in private practice, a community health center, or a hospital would act as a gatekeeper, manage all of a patient's care, and serve as a financial manager of a set budget to cover the patient's medical needs.

Although its primary motivation was to ensure access to care for the poor, the program had cost implications, especially for the states, which share the cost of Medicaid with the federal government. It set out to cut costs by capitalizing on managed care's developing track record in holding the line and by strengthening the ability of community health centers to withstand competition from private insurers.

"There was a sense that state Medicaid budgets were rising at the time, and that the states were concerned," said Alan Cohen, the Foundation vice president who oversaw the external evaluation of this initiative. "If HMOs could be shown to be more cost constraining, you might be able to kill two birds with one stone—improving access to routine primary care for people who can't get it in urban and rural settings and providing care at lower cost than Medicaid fee-for-service. It might relieve some of the budget pressures at the state level."

The evaluation found that the program did reduce utilization and costs, and some health centers that participated in the program still use this approach today, said Drew Altman, who shepherded the program when he was a Foundation vice president. "This was the first really big effort to support Medicaid managed care, and it did some good," Altman said. "This program pioneered some of the early models of Medicaid managed care—who's going to do it and how you do it. We wanted to safely control Medicaid costs without losing benefits and to help safety-net institutions to be players in managed care so they weren't cut out by the private insurance companies."

### *The Faculty Fellowships in Health Care Finance Program*

Another initiative with a broader purpose that contained a cost control element was the Faculty Fellowships in Health Care Finance program, a $5.1 million initiative that began in 1984 and continued through 1992. During the first year of the fellowship, the fellows studied at the Johns Hopkins University and were placed in a relevant organization, such as a health insurer or a government health care financing agency. The second year, they returned to their university positions, receiving a stipend to conduct research on health care financing. In this way, the program would fund the training of academics who would then become experts in the revolutionary changes under way in how health care was being financed. "We hoped we would turn out a generation of people with good economic credentials interested in applied policy in health care economics," said Bruce Vladeck, who was a Foundation assistant vice president when the program was being planned.

But the program did not perform up to expectations, an evaluation found. There was disagreement about the goals of the program and the kinds of participants it was supposed to attract. Moreover, the evaluation found that many of the participants were not as "distinguished" as the Foundation had hoped they would be; for their part, many of the fellows were dissatisfied with the program, finding it wasn't "compelling" enough and didn't fill the gaps in their knowledge. The program was also faulted for not recruiting candidates aggressively enough.

"The big disappointment was that most of the fellows didn't have an impact when they returned to their schools or weren't likely to have," said Alan Cohen. "It wasn't an effective program." The Faculty Fellowships in Health Care Finance program was not refunded, but in 1992 the Foundation did launch two companion programs—Scholars in Health Policy Research and Investigator Awards in Health Policy Research—that focus more broadly on health policy issues.[6]

### Changes in Health Care Financing and Organization

One last outgrowth of the Foundation's 1980s funding of cost containment initiatives was the Program for Research and Development on Health Care Costs, later to be modified and retitled the Program for Demonstration and Research on Health Care Costs. The original emphasis was on new approaches to cutting health care costs, and grantees were funded to do research, demonstrations, or evaluations.

From 1982 to 1987, some forty-six grants costing $10.6 million were made under the umbrella of this program. Although many of the projects were worthwhile, the Foundation concluded that they would have been far more useful if they had not focused solely on cost, while ignoring the major changes and policy issues dominating the health care marketplace.

In 1988, reflecting the growth in the Foundation's own understanding of the complexity of health policy issues, the program was retooled and renamed Changes in Health Care Financing and Organization, or HCFO. The nation's largest private investigator-initiated grant program, HCFO provides funds for research, demonstration projects, and evaluations that look at the many emerging approaches for financing and organizing the health care delivery system and how they might affect access, quality, and cost. Through mid-June 2003, 192 awards totaling $55.8 million had been made under HCFO.

Managed by AcademyHealth, a Washington, D.C.–based nonprofit health services research and policy organization, HCFO has become a resource for both policymakers and researchers. "Our significant contribution is probably in part understanding how various public and private strategies people have devised have worked," said Anne Gauthier, HCFO program director and AcademyHealth vice president. "This includes such work as looking at the impact of managed care, insurance market reform, and studies that look at the behavioral response of key players when you put in cost containment strategies, with managed care being a huge one among them."

An outside evaluation of HCFO done in 2002 by Jack Hoadley and Michael Gluck at Georgetown University found that its "projects address some of the most important health policy issues being debated at the national and state levels" and cited its work on insurance market reform, physician payment, hospital financing, cost containment, the uninsured, and risk adjustment. Many HCFO grantees are highly regarded within their fields and looked to by public policymakers, the authors said.

Former Foundation president Schroeder cited as particularly "promising" HCFO's many studies looking at the concept of risk adjustment, in which managed care health insurers carrying a heavier load of sick patients are paid more for covering them and thus have an incentive to provide them with quality care. Currently, the best way for an insurance company to keep costs down is to avoid insuring sick people, who need more care and thus cost it more. Risk adjustment realigns payments from within a health plan pool or employer plan, allocating more to an insurer with more high-risk patients—and thus equalizing financial risk. This would give insurers a monetary incentive to enroll patients with high risk factors. Although risk adjustment has begun to be used in the public sector, particularly in the Medicare + Choice program, it has not yet gained wide acceptance among private insurers.

HCFO was one of the early movers in risk adjustment, having funded some of the first research aimed at developing tools for assessing what a health insurer's risk would be and then running simulations to show how the assessment tools might work in practice. HCFO also funded demonstrations of risk adjustment tools within the Medicaid program. And through its research and conferences, it has shown that although assessing risk is highly complex and requires a great deal of data, the tool doesn't have to be perfect to be useful.

Of particular note has been the work of Richard Kronick of the University of California, San Diego, and Harold Luft of the University of California, San Francisco. Kronick developed a risk adjustment payment system that provides Medicaid managed care plans with a rich enough payment to cover the costs of patients who are sicker or have disabilities. A number of states use this system with their Medicaid managed care programs. Luft has been designing a user-friendly Web-based tool for potential use by actuaries or health consultants to test which of many risk adjustment models would work best in different situations.

Despite HCFO's having funded a great deal of research on health financing, organization, and costs, the program is not without its critics. One of them is former Health Care Financing Administration chief Bruce Vladeck. "They do an amazing job of following every short-term fad in academic health policy and have helped reinforce whatever the conventional wisdom was at any point in time rather than calling it into question," he said recently. He cited as an example "tons of research" that HCFO had supported on refining methods of providing financial incentives for physicians in managed care plans. "This was the hottest thing in academic health economics," he said. "But when people started doing it in the real world, many doctors didn't understand it and gave up."

On the whole, though, HCFO is generally well regarded. "This program . . . is seen as an important source of funding not found elsewhere," the evaluators wrote. "Federal funders are less interested in organization and financing than in quality of care and mandated studies. In addition, federal resources are becoming more constrained."

## —ᜃᜃ— Postscript

Surely health care costs will continue to rise, but why should they concern us so? "This is something that matters to us if it's not fair," former Foundation president Steven Schroeder said. "It matters if costs keep people from getting things that are vital for their health and well-being. It matters if costs exacerbate distributional issues that aren't fair. It matters if costs push a nation into investing less wisely for its overall economic health."

Over twenty-two years—or longer, according to some viewpoints—the Foundation has tried to find solutions to this stubborn problem, first through cost containment initiatives and then through more sophisticated approaches that examine how the health care delivery system is paid for and organized.

It has found no prescription pill that will lower health insurance bills or the nation's overall spending. Instead, the Foundation has learned some basic lessons about both cost containment and itself.

"In some ways, it's misleadingly simple—the idea of cost control seems so straightforward, but we've found that it's actually very complex," said the Foundation's Robert Hughes. "It gets at every aspect of health care delivery. And there is no quick fix that even a majority of a minority would go for. It's not clear what to do."

The Robert Wood Johnson Foundation has learned to scale back its aspirations for what it can do—through conferences, research, demonstrations, and evaluations, it can stimulate debate and contribute knowledge and analysis that may lead to important, though more modest, changes in health care policy.

According to the Kaiser Family Foundation's Drew Altman, it's a matter of gaining perspective. "A foundation has to be realistic about what it can do in a $1.4 trillion dollar national health care system," Altman said. "You have to understand how marginal you are but wake up raring to go because you have a role to play. Foundations can be a bit player in the big game or a major player at the margins. Most choose the latter."

Today the Foundation's continuing but indirect commitment to cost containment can be seen primarily in its HCFO program, the Center for Studying Health System Change's reports on health care costs, and various individual grants addressing health system policy research. The Foundation's new president and chief executive officer, Risa Lavizzo-Mourey, expects one cost-related area of study to be evaluating the defined contribution model—also called "consumer-driven health care." This is hailed by some as a way to give employees incentives to manage their own health care more cost-efficiently by providing them a set sum of money to use as they wish for their care along with an insurance plan with a high deductible.

The new Foundation chief, who took the helm as the country again was wrestling with stratospheric health care costs and double-digit premium hikes, expresses a clear-eyed view about what the past tells the Foundation about what it can do. "We can have an impact in defining and identifying new models, evaluating solutions that are put in place," Lavizzo-Mourey said. "We are not likely to implement large-scale change. We have a role to seek information and try to evaluate various techniques that might be useful in forming new models. We don't have a regulatory role or really strong leverage in reducing costs."

## Notes

1. "Goals Update." In *Annual Report.* The Robert Wood Johnson Foundation, 1996, p. 29.
2. In the spring of 2003, the goal was modified slightly to reflect the importance of high-quality, not just basic, health care. The new goal is "To assure that all Americans have access to quality health care at a reasonable cost."
3. Brown, L. D., and McLaughlin, C. "Constraining Costs at the Community Level: A Critique." *Health Affairs,* 1990, *9*(4), 6–28.
4. Schroeder, S. A., Cohen, A., and Cantor, J. "Perspectives: The Funders." *Health Affairs,* 1990, *9*(4), 29–33.
5. Dunlop, J., and Stiles, G. "Perspectives: A Local Program Director and a National Advisory Chairman." *Health Affairs,* 1990, *9*(4), 42–46.
6. For a discussion of the Faculty Fellowships in Health Care Finance, the Scholars in Health Policy Research, and the Investigator Awards in Health Policy Research programs, see Colby, D. C. "Building Health Policy Research Capacity in the Social Sciences." In *To Improve Health and Health Care, Vol. VI: The Robert Wood Johnson Foundation Anthology.* San Francisco: Jossey-Bass, 2003.

# The Teaching Nursing Home Program

*Ethan Bronner*

---

## Editors' Introduction

In most cases, the chapters of The Robert Wood Johnson Foundation *Anthology* focus on recently or nearly completed activities. In this way, we are able to provide timely reports of emerging findings. Every year, however, at least one chapter takes a look back at a long-finished program; this allows us to assess outcomes through a longer lens. This year, the *Anthology* looks back on the Teaching Nursing Home Program, an effort the Foundation funded between 1982 and 1987 to improve the quality of nursing home care and the clinical training of nurses by linking nursing schools with nursing homes.

The program was based on the model of educating physicians whereby medical residents get on-the-job training by caring for patients in teaching hospitals. If this model enhanced the skills of young physicians and improved the care of patients, why, Foundation staff members asked, wouldn't the same be true if nursing students received on-the-job training in nursing homes?

As told by *New York Times* editor and frequent *Anthology* contributor Ethan Bronner, the story of the Teaching Nursing Home Program is not one of a uniformly successful initiative. Maintaining relationships between nursing schools and nursing homes turned out to be more difficult than expected; nursing homes had less money than did hospitals; and geriatrics was not an attractive field for many new nurses. Although the program's use of quantitative measures contributed to later evaluations of home health agencies' performance and many of the program's alumnae attained great stature in the nursing profession, teaching nursing homes are today the exception rather than the norm.

While teaching nursing homes may no longer be a priority of the Foundation, its interest in nursing and in services for the elderly continues. The Foundation has $173 million in active grants aimed at strengthening the delivery of care for chronically ill individuals, a large proportion of whom are elderly. And improving the quality of the nursing workforce and of nursing services is one of the eight Foundation priority areas that the board of trustees adopted in January 2003.

~m~ I n 1980, Bruce Vladeck shook the nation when he published his book *Unloving Care: The Nursing Home Tragedy,* which chronicled government failure and rapacious private profiteering in an industry that had exploded during the 1960s.[1] With Americans living longer and increasingly spending time in nursing homes of widely varying quality, the book called for a restructuring of care for the elderly.

The Robert Wood Johnson Foundation was eager to play a role, and from 1982 through 1987 funded the Teaching Nursing Home Program. Inspired by the success of teaching hospitals, the program aimed at improving nursing home care by linking the homes with nearby schools of nursing. The five-year, $6.7 million program sought to teach nursing students hands-on geriatrics while bringing rigor and research to the nursing homes.

The Teaching Nursing Home Program was modest by Foundation standards and, at best, was also modest in outcome. Some consider it to have been a failure. Launched in the Foundation's classic style as a pilot, with the hope that it would be picked up and replicated by other foundations or the federal government, or both, the Teaching Nursing Home Program ended with no takers at the time and was not renewed by The Robert Wood Johnson Foundation. Of the eleven schools of nursing and the dozen nursing homes from around the country that participated in the program, none directly follow the model anymore. As Patricia Patrizi, a former assistant director of the program and now an evaluation consultant to foundations, put it, "It was a model based on improved medical care when what was really needed was improved social care. This was a time when cost containment was central in health care, and the program advocated a kind of Cadillac model that was bound to fail."

Alan Cohen, a professor of health policy and management at Boston University and a former vice president at The Robert Wood Johnson Foundation in the 1980s, said the program had little impact on the field, adding, "I think it comes down to one fundamental question that always is raised when you talk about a new approach to health care delivery: Who is going to pay for it? Where will the money come from so there will be incentives for more nursing homes to adopt the model? Frankly, I don't think there was clear-cut evidence that would have suggested to payers such as the Health Care Financing Administration (now the Centers for Medicare & Medicaid Services) and state Medicaid programs that this was really worth replicating."

Yet in the field of geriatric nursing, the Teaching Nursing Home Program is honored as a pioneer. While it is viewed as a program that suffered from unfulfilled promise, it is also viewed as a program that made a difference in a number of areas. For example, the concept of linking research and nurse training with nursing homes remains alive in a nation where the very old are the fastest-growing segment of our population. There are, today, several new teaching nursing home programs on university campuses in places like Lubbock, Texas, and Lexington, Kentucky. Their administrators say they were inspired by the first program. In addition, there are nearly six thousand nurse practitioners—registered nurses with advanced degrees—in geriatrics, 80 percent of whom work in nursing homes, and such a development was one of the program's aims. Those nurse practitioners gather data on such factors as pressure sores and incontinence using the methods developed by Peter Shaughnessy, a professor of geriatric medicine at the University of Colorado Health Sciences Center and one of the leaders of the program evaluation team, among others. Nursing students at many schools, which have historically offered no exposure to geriatrics, now spend at least a small portion of their training in that area. This is not solely a direct result of the Teaching Nursing Home Program, of course, but the program is often cited when the training is discussed. Home health care for the elderly, which has exploded in importance, is now often judged and rated using approaches developed by Shaughnessy and based partly on his work in the program. Finally, a core of geriatric nursing specialists who launched the Teaching Nursing Home Program have fanned out to hospitals, nursing schools, and nursing associations, and continue to spread the techniques, the results, and the spirit of the pilot program.

"There is no poster child for the elderly in our society," observed Marla Salmon, dean of the Nell Hodgson Woodruff School of Nursing at Emory University in Atlanta and a trustee of The Robert Wood Johnson

Foundation, in reflecting on why programs like the one for teaching nursing homes did not enjoy wide support. "We are ambivalent about nursing homes because they remind us of our vulnerability. The Teaching Nursing Home Program was fundamental, however—a paradigm shift. It sought to operationalize care for the elderly, and it provided a model for improving health care in nursing homes that is still widely discussed."

Although Emory was not one of the eleven participants in the program, it is one of the beneficiaries because it has set up a program based on the model. All Emory nursing students put in some time at one of two nursing homes on campus—something their predecessors twenty years ago did not do—and Emory has become a center for innovative geriatric care. At the A. G. Rhodes Nursing Home in Wesley Woods, Jennifer Reardon, a nursing student who plans to go into pediatrics, spent two days working with what are today often called "maturing adults," meaning the aged. In the shining, welcoming chambers of the nursing home, Reardon helped a one-hundred-year-old resident with exercises by placing weights on her feet and arms and attending to her other needs. Reardon's supervisor was Jean Pals, a nurse-educator with the division of geriatric medicine at Emory University.

During a break, Pals discussed with Reardon and two other students the differences between treating a thirty-five-year-old and an eighty-five-year-old. One is likely to have a strong family support system, the other is not; one is likely to have a strong immune system, the other is not; one is likely to go home after the treatment, the other may already be home. None of the students training under Pals that day planned to be a geriatric nurse. But they are still young and focused on the problems of youth. Nobody, Pals says, is born to geriatrics. Nonetheless, even their brief exposure opened a world to them. One day, when they are older, their interest in the aged may well increase.

"Like most students, I had the image that a nursing home was a place where people go to die," remarked Camille Louisy-Oladele, who was training with Reardon. "It's smelly and people can't walk and all you do is go around changing bedpans. Now I see that it doesn't have to be that way, that there are people who get better and who do leave. And we also see what kind of difference we can make in a place like this."

Emory is one of the few facilities (though their numbers are grow-ing) in the country where no physical restraints are used on residents. As explained by Dr. Ted Johnson, director of the Atlanta VA Medical Cen-ter Nursing Home Care Unit and assistant professor of medicine at Emory University School of Medicine, in the past nursing homes have often been places where residents sat in diapers, tied down through restraint vests. Now the beds in his facility do not even have simple bars.

This is partly due to the work of Elizabeth Capezuti, who until re-cently held the Wesley Woods Chair in Gerontological Nursing at Emory. Capezuti, who emerged from the Teaching Nursing Home Program group in the 1980s, focuses her research on how to increase the dignity and the comfort of nursing home residents. She has been working with bed man-ufacturers to improve the way nursing home beds function. Through the Emory Center for Health in Aging, she has also focused on patient falls. Working with Dr. Joseph Ouslander, the founding director of the center, Capezuti helped develop a program for resident safety, within a so-called culture of safety. Since there are today more nursing home beds in the United States than hospital beds, and since those over age eighty-five make up the fastest-growing segment of the American population, such re-thinking of nursing home care is vital. It is a shift anticipated by those who conceived the Teaching Nursing Home Program two decades ago, when few others were as focused on the care and health of aging people as they are today.

## —ᴡᴡ— The Birth of the Teaching Nursing Home Program

The idea of a teaching nursing home came from Linda Aiken, who ar-rived at The Robert Wood Johnson Foundation in 1974 as a program officer after having been a postdoctoral fellow at the University of Wisconsin–Madison. From the start of her career, she had been interested in the evolving professional roles of nurses and their connections with pa-tient outcomes. She was struck by the growing number of nursing home scandals and the clear need for high-level care in these homes. They may be called "nursing" homes, she noticed, but nursing was not their strength.

With nursing homes becoming such a growing part of the health care picture—their numbers doubled from thirteen thousand in 1963 to nearly twenty-six thousand in 1982—she asked herself how to improve them.

Given Aiken's background—a nurse who had gone back to school for a master's degree and a doctorate—she thought the way to fix the problem might be to build links between nursing schools and nursing homes. She drew inspiration from a similar and successful arrangement during the 1960s involving public and veterans' hospitals on the one hand and medical schools on the other.

"Back in the 1960s, there was an acknowledgment that public hospitals and those of the Veterans Administration (now the Department of Veterans Affairs) were substandard," Aiken recalled. "They couldn't get good doctors and nurses, and they were filled with scandals. The solution that was found was to affiliate those hospitals with medical schools and teaching hospitals. It was a highly successful plan. Today many VA and public hospitals are as good as any in the country."

Aiken asked herself why the same would not work for nursing homes. Most such homes really had no capacity for providing therapeutic care, and so doctors had no real interest in working there. She figured that if nurses could be brought in, doctors might be more willing to join them. That might reduce some of the problems, like bedsores and routine dispatch to hospital emergency rooms that cause disruption and discomfort for the residents.

Another factor in nursing homes had drawn her attention. It was becoming increasingly clear that such facilities had two very different sets of residents—long-term ones and those who would leave after some weeks or months. A 1976 paper of which she was coauthor in the *Journal of the American Geriatrics Society* found that 43 percent of nursing home residents stayed for less than six months.[2]

There was also another issue—what Aiken considered the worrying isolation of academic nursing from real care. She thought nursing education would be dramatically improved through an association with nursing homes and suspected that the more manageable size of nursing homes would be easier for the nurses than huge hospitals.

## —ɯ— The Program in Operation

Having gained the approval of The Robert Wood Johnson Foundation's board, Aiken and her colleagues set up the program, which was cosponsored by the American Academy of Nursing and administered by the University of Pennsylvania's School of Nursing. Fifty-three schools applied to participate in the program, and eleven were accepted. They were Georgetown University and Catholic University in Washington, D.C.; the State University of New York at Binghamton; Rutgers University in Newark, New Jersey; the University of Wisconsin in Madison; Case Western Reserve in Cleveland; the University of Cincinnati; Rush-Presbyterian–St. Luke's Medical Center in Chicago; Creighton University in Omaha, Nebraska; the University of Utah in Salt Lake City; and Oregon Health & Science University in Portland. Each school chose one nursing home affiliate except Creighton, which chose two. The projects had varying start-up dates in 1982. Each nursing school had a slightly different history and status. Five were privately endowed, six publicly funded. All offered a graduate program in nursing. Six of the graduate programs offered a major in gerontological nursing (one was a geropsychiatric program), and three offered a subspecialty or minor in it. Before the Teaching Nursing Home Program, all but two of the schools had some formal or informal agreement with their affiliated nursing homes for clinical placement of students.

The twelve nursing homes that participated were also diverse, but had one trait in common: they provided a higher than average level of care. Some were recognized leaders in their areas. All except one were nonprofit. Eight were freestanding, four hospital-based.

The program's administrators at the University of Pennsylvania School of Nursing set objectives for four areas: to increase quality of care; to increase interest in geriatrics at the school of nursing; to improve staff development; and to ensure financial survival beyond Foundation funding. Each pairing of school and nursing home outlined strategies in all four areas.

The main aim in quality of care was to improve the physical and psychological well-being of residents. There were programs in bladder and bowel training to combat incontinence, a skin care program to reduce the number and severity of decubitus ulcers, or bedsores, and activities to prevent falls and monitor drug use. Many programs entailed rewriting nursing protocols and developing interdisciplinary approaches to care. In one case, a registered nurse assumed twenty-four-hour responsibility for a group of residents. On the psychosocial side, group activities for residents were developed. Three projects formed residents' councils to advocate for residents' rights and to increase participation. An additional goal was to decrease the rate at which residents were sent to emergency rooms and outside hospitals. While this became important for residents, it proved to be less so for the nursing homes. In many cases, nursing homes are reimbursed by Medicaid for "bed holds"—that is, for a portion of the time a resident is hospitalized—thereby actually giving them an incentive to use emergency rooms more, not less.

The goals of increasing interest in geriatrics at the schools of nursing and improving staff development were to be met by adding faculty members trained in gerontology, stepping up research in the field, and building the number of students ultimately interested in going into it. Some projects offered adjunct or clinical faculty appointments to nursing home staff members (although in many cases, staff members lacked the needed academic degrees to qualify). As Joy Smith, the recently retired director of nursing at the Providence Benedictine Nursing Center in Mount Angel, Oregon, put it while the program was going on, "This forces the staff to reexamine their practices because they are demonstrating them for students. I hear staff saying, 'The students are coming and we have to watch our procedures.'"[3] Since one of the biggest problems of nursing homes is frequent staff turnover, an important goal regarding staff development was retention. One indirect path toward this was staff training and development as well as career counseling. The theory was that increasing staff knowledge and skill would lead to greater job satisfaction.

To help the program survive beyond the years of the pilot project, negotiations were begun with state agencies. Calculations were made on how to share costs between the nursing homes and the schools. In a few cases, participants were able to increase the Medicaid reimbursement rate for their nursing home affiliate by demonstrating improved care.

No pilot project is ever easy, but from the outset the Teaching Nursing Home Program ran into difficulties. The first might best be described as a culture gap between the academic nursing schools and the more rough-and-ready nursing homes. Nursing home staff often seemed to resent the outsiders, viewing them as intruders who thought they knew better and who were going to create unnecessary work. Meanwhile, many faculty members were typically unfamiliar with the regulatory difficulties in nursing homes and the small profit margin on which they operated. Relations eased after the first year or two in most cases and were even harmonious in some cases.

A second problem was frequent staff turnover. One teaching nursing home had six different administrators over three years, while another had four. Many others had at least one change at the top. Each new arrival needed to be oriented to the project. Joint appointments also proved complicated, since many nursing home staff members did not have the needed academic credentials for even adjunct appointments. Moreover, the nursing professors found that their heavy clinical responsibilities at the nursing homes conflicted with their need to pursue teaching and research for tenure. In addition, many of the faculty members had nine-month appointments at the school, whereas their nursing home responsibilities were for a twelve-month year.

Ultimately, The Robert Wood Johnson Foundation did not renew the five-year grant. "We needed another four to five years of funding," says Mathy Mezey, who was the director of the program at the University of Pennsylvania, where she was also a professor of nursing. She now runs the John A. Hartford Institute for Geriatric Nursing at New York University. "If we had gotten it, we would have helped to stabilize good partnerships. We would have positioned them more centrally in their communities. We also tried, but failed, to get several states to have several nursing homes as models for the state."

Many foundation grants are not renewed. In this case, a combination of skepticism toward the model and changes within The Robert Wood Johnson Foundation itself were the likely cause. David Rogers, the president, left, and many of those closest to him who followed him out the door, including vice presidents Linda Aiken and Robert Blendon, were among the program's biggest supporters. Former Foundation vice president Alan Cohen points out that by the late 1980s, The Robert Wood Johnson Foundation was seeking to move support services for the frail elderly out of institutions and into the community. He also felt that tacking the evaluation onto the project later, rather than making it an integral part from the beginning, may have undermined the program's chances for demonstrating success.

Other factors in the late 1980s clearly didn't help. The nation was entering a period of economic recession. Managed care was settling into the health industry, leading to severe cost cutting. There was also another in a series of periodic nurse shortages. And despite increased attention to gerontology, it was still a stepchild in the health field. Sources of support for faculty members at nursing schools also began to shift, making them more grant dependent. And while geriatric nurse practitioners began to be reimbursed through Medicare for their work in skilled nursing facilities at a rate of 85 percent of that of physicians, Medicaid remained the main source of funds for most nursing homes. Teaching nursing homes did not offer Medicaid ways to cut its costs.

## —ɯ— The Rutgers College of Nursing's Experience

In many ways, the experience at Rutgers was emblematic of the program.[4] The Rutgers College of Nursing originally chose two county nursing homes to be its partners—the Long-Term Care Division of Bergen Pines County Hospital in Paramus and a second home that was on the verge of decertification. But as the program was about to start, it became clear that including the second home was not feasible. It was dropped. Bergen Pines was a large facility with 571 beds, located on a 1,300-bed campus in an affluent suburb in northern New Jersey. It had established a name for itself as a leader in nursing care.

Lucille Joel, professor and director of clinical affairs at the Rutgers College of Nursing, was chosen to run the program, and one of the conditions imposed on the nursing home was that she serve as one of its two associate directors. This was the only case in the program where a faculty member was given direct authority rather than an advisory role in the home. Joel recalls that while Rutgers chose Bergen Pines for its quality, what she and others saw when they entered the facility was well below their expectations.

"There were more urinary catheters than there should have been, more bowel problems, more bedsores, more people dependent on nurses' aides for eating," she said. "We also had not been prepared for how difficult many of the cases were. The residents were more disabled, more compromised than those in private sector homes, yet the reimbursement was the same as in those other homes. That actually led us to work with the county on a class action suit to get the state of New Jersey to increase reimbursement to the county homes. We were able to get more reimbursement per day for the county homes." That led to an additional $1.5 million coming to the home.

There were other accomplishments. Just two faculty members were involved in gerontological nursing in early 1982, but the number rose to six in 1983 and to twelve in 1986. In addition, some twenty-nine student and faculty research projects in gerontology were completed during the project, and twenty-five publications were produced. Among the research projects was the development of an instrument to diagnose depression in the nonverbal elderly.

The project's leaders realized within a year, however, that their clinical proposal was too ambitious. It was nearly impossible to have an impact on all 571 residents at one time. As a result, two residential units of sixty beds each were set apart from the rest of the home to serve as experimental centers. Once strategies there proved effective, they were to be moved out beyond the units to the entire nursing home. One problem with that approach was that it took away the possibility of comparing the results at Bergen Pines with other nursing homes used as control groups, which had been the original intent of the evaluation.

Within the first year of the program, clinical results were persuasive in the 120 experimental beds. Among the residents in those beds, there was a 50 percent decrease in bedsores, a 23 percent decrease in the use of physical restraints in one unit, a 25 percent decrease in the use of enemas, and 18 percent fewer acute care transfers than in the previous year. Such results were typical of many other participants in the Teaching Nursing Home Program.[5]

By the end of the second year, there was a further 7 percent decrease in bedsores, 10 percent less use of physical restraints, 13 percent less incontinence, and 17 percent fewer residents on psychotropic drugs. Similar results were found in the following two years.

But by early 1987 nearly all the documented gains either had begun to reverse or were entirely reversed. For example, in 1987 barely more than 6 percent of the residents were able to feed themselves, compared with 27 percent in 1986. The use of physical restraints had increased to 75 percent, compared with 59 percent in 1986 and 64 percent in 1985.[6]

What led to the decline? It is hard to say, but it may have had to do with a decision by the county administration to award a management contract to an investor-owned corporation in the hope of reversing long-standing deficits. Nonprofessionals were substituted for licensed nurses as positions opened. The new managers also declined to give Rutgers faculty members an equal role in running the facility. As Lucille Joel recalled later, "When the corporation came in, they cut us off from information and instituted their own changes, including reducing registered nurses and other key personnel. They refused to listen to us about anything."

Rutgers withdrew from Bergen Pines, choosing to finish up its Teaching Nursing Home Program years working with the Daughters of Miriam Center for the Aged in Clifton, an eight-hundred-bed religiously affiliated home with multiple levels of care. Rutgers faculty members did not have any direct control over this home. Their role was purely advisory, focusing on areas of staff development, quality assurance, research, and long-term planning and programming. That relationship continued for a decade.

Although other participants in the Teaching Nursing Home Program did not face such a rupture with their homes, the Rutgers experience exemplifies the program's fortunes. There were, as in most of the nursing homes, tough relations at first, followed by encouraging results, good clinical research, and increased involvement in gerontology on the part of nursing students and faculty. Nonetheless, the project was unable to demonstrate that it could be a money saver for homes that operate on narrow margins. And the link between college and nursing home was an often difficult and ultimately unsuccessful one.

As Joel summed it up, "From the beginning of the Rutgers program, nothing was easy." Contract negotiation was beset by a series of misunderstandings and deficiencies in the art of compromise on the part of both institutions. The academic interests of faculty members predominated over any responsibility for clinical care, and administrators in the home were hesitant to give any authority to individuals who were external to their own system. Only mutual respect and trust between nursing leaders in both arenas allowed the basic philosophy of the project to prevail and to find permanent protection in the resulting affiliation agreement.

One account of the Rutgers experience noted lack of mutual trust, but pointed out other obstacles: "The lingering mistrust between education and service and the hurdles of contract negotiation that this created seem small compared to the entrenched attitudes toward the aged, most particularly the institutionalized aged. Undergraduate students were less than exuberant about a clinical placement in the home. Staff members were blind to the fact that there could be more quality of life for residents, and proceeded with their usual infantilizing approaches to care."[7]

In conclusion, Joel said that change was "slow but glorious" and would have continued if there had not been a rupture with the new management. "Experience with clinical programs, staffing, and resident classification systems reinforced the conviction that there were models for care of the institutionalized, frail elderly that we had yet to explore," she said.

## —ɯ— Evaluation of the Program

That is how many people involved in the Teaching Nursing Home Program felt when it was over—that it had been reasonably successful for both home and college and had opened vistas onto new areas and methods in the expanding field of gerontology. But since the program had not been renewed, it was unable to fulfill its potential. Others were far more skeptical of its value. Some nursing home staff members and outside evaluators considered the program flawed in concept and the wrong model for the field.

The program did show signs of success, but in a somewhat less clearcut fashion than its advocates had hoped. And given the costs involved in maintaining such a program, the likelihood that it could serve as a model nationally was bleak. This is mainly because evaluation of the project could not be systematic, since it was added after the project had begun.

This meant that the collection of baseline data was done retrospectively and often incompletely, and the use of control group nursing homes, against which the results of changes that had taken place within the program sites could be compared, was partial.

Peter Shaughnessy and Andrew Kramer of the University of Colorado Health Sciences Center were chosen to be the program's evaluators. Beginning their work in late 1983, after the Teaching Nursing Home Program had been going for a year, they were given an advisory committee of other evaluators whom the Foundation had turned down for the grant. This made for some unusual tensions. And they were urged to look only at what they called the "big picture"—functional change and hospitalization rates—and not to get bogged down in clinical details.

Their advisory committee and the federal government's Health Care Financing Administration, which was brought in as a cofunder of the evaluation, were most focused on reduced hospitalization and increased rehabilitation. But Shaughnessy and Kramer worried that neither category would produce clean results. Moreover, when rehabilitation among the frail elderly occurs, it is not easily attributed to any one factor. So the evaluators pushed to expand the sources of evaluation by gathering data on less spectacular matters such as urinary tract infection, congestive heart failure, and distribution of psychotropic drugs. They were worried that the program's virtues would not be evident from research based purely on the so-called big questions. As Kramer put it, "We were concerned that you might not be able to make the bedridden walk with a teaching nursing home."[8]

The evaluators found six nursing homes located in the same states as those of the Teaching Nursing Home Program that had similar traits and compared them with six of the program participants. This was fine as far as it went, but it created some problems. First, it meant that the six other program nursing homes were not evaluated with the same care. In addition, baseline data were collected only retrospectively from nursing home records and were not as comprehensive or as exact as the data obtained during the intervention period.

As Alan Cohen, who arrived at The Robert Wood Johnson Foundation in late 1984, put it, "When they brought the evaluators in well after the beginning of the implementation of the program, they put them in a really tough position. There was a tendency on the part of many of the evaluators to try to use process measures as proxies for some of the outcomes. Because the evaluation budget was constrained, they couldn't go out and collect primary data to get at some of those outcome questions that the Foundation staff wanted answered."

The data that the evaluators did collect were impressive. Hospitalization rates in the first three months—meaning the chance of a resident being sent to a hospital at least once within three months of arrival—were different between the two groups of homes. There was a drop of 7 percent among the experimental group compared with an increase of 4.9 percent in the control group. That makes a mean difference of 11.9 percent. That pattern continued throughout the first year, although it was more pronounced for short-stay and Medicare patients than for long-stay and Medicaid patients. There was also a significant drop in the number of days spent in the hospital by the Teaching Nursing Home Program residents, down from 3 days to 1 day over six months and from 3.4 days to 1.3 days over twelve months.[9] The two main reasons for the decline in hospitalization were thought to be programs that enhanced or stabilized activities of daily living and the involvement of nurses in the planning of care.

There were also 20 percent fewer bedsores in the teaching nursing homes than in the control homes and a 22 percent reduction in bowel incontinence, as well as marked improvements in stabilization of bathing and ambulation. Physical restraint was down, as was the use of psychotropic medication. As the evaluators wrote in a 1995 review, "nursing home quality improvement through affiliation with schools of nursing is possible and warrants consideration on a more widespread basis."[10]

Mathy Mezey, the program's former director, said the hope was that all these data showing improvements would lead to the spread of the program. "We all hoped, certainly, that the model of the teaching nursing home would be a sustaining one and be encouraged in a number of ways; and that the states would designate certain teaching nursing homes, the federal government would grant some waivers for teaching nursing homes, and the industry itself would see the advantages," she said. "None of that was really accomplished within the five years of the project."

Peter Shaughnessy, a leader of the evaluation team, said that in retrospect more should have been made of the program's success so that Congress and the federal government would take up the program where The Robert Wood Johnson Foundation left it. "Whose job is it to take the bit in their teeth and run with it on this program from the standpoint of its national value?" he asked. "We didn't see it as our job. Now that I look back on it, I can kick myself—even though we didn't have funding to do any more—for not trying to squeak out more at the margin in order to better communicate the message, 'OK, health care society, this is important, don't overlook it' and in a constructive way beat people over the head with the fact that you can't overlook this."

Joan Lynaugh, associate director of the program at the University of Pennsylvania School of Nursing and now a retired professor of nursing, said the project was probably a long shot from the start. "We tried to convince policymakers that this would make care cheaper, but that was hard to demonstrate," she said. "On the other side, we were trying to drag schools of nursing into this by bribing them and then making a big fuss over the results. The faculty were uninterested and unmotivated. It was hard to get them to redirect their interests and carve out space in the curriculum. Gerontology has never been as sexy as critical care or oncology nursing."

Patricia Patrizi, the former assistant director of the project, said that improving health care in nursing homes was not the main problem, since so many nursing home residents are demented. "You are really talking about maintenance," she said. "It doesn't take a whole lot to improve bedsores. It is simply about moving people. The key is inclusion of family and improved social setting."

## —॥॥— The Program in Retrospect

Interestingly, although funding for the Teaching Nursing Home Program stopped over ten years ago, geriatric nurse specialists continue to recall it with pride. May Wykle, dean of the Frances Payne Bolton School of Nursing at Case Western Reserve University, said her school no longer had a program link with the nursing home—the Margaret Wagner House, now called the Kethley House—but that it continues to have a formal affiliation agreement, and both undergraduate and graduate nursing students have clinical experiences there.

Wykle, who was the site's project director under the Teaching Nursing Home Program, believes that the nursing home was improved by the school's involvement with it two decades ago. "The end result of the Teaching Nursing Home Program was that we improved the quality of care there, and it is now considered one of the best nursing homes in the Cleveland area," she said.

Others disagree, however, saying that the nursing home had been a top facility before the involvement of her faculty. In any case, nursing students continue to train at the home—something they did not do before the program.

Today there is a growing group of researchers focused on the needs of the elderly, people like twenty-seven-year-old Laura Wagner, who emerged in some sense from the Teaching Nursing Home Program environment. Wagner is working toward a Ph.D. in nursing at Emory University after studying for her registered nursing degree at Case Western and becoming a nurse practitioner at Penn. Wagner worked as a nurse practitioner at a nursing home in Columbus, Ohio, and helped change the way emergency room transfers were carried out there. Now, for her doctorate, she is focusing on falls in nursing homes. Her mentors are largely graduates of the Teaching Nursing Home Program.

Some involved in care for the elderly believe the Teaching Nursing Home Program was one factor that helped focus attention on a series of quality-of-care issues like bedsores, incontinence, safety, mental health, and the use of physical restraints. Today some of the nursing homes formerly involved in the program are moving to a restraint-free environment. That is the case at Kethley House, according to May Wykle.

Another change to which the program contributed is the increased use of nurse practitioners in nursing homes. Debbie Gunter, who works for UnitedHealthcare, which owns Evercare, is part of a group of 40 nurse practitioners who cover a set of nursing homes in the Atlanta area. Evercare started in Minnesota, spread to more than a dozen states, and now has 350 nurse practitioners working around the country. Gunter says that she and her colleagues collect data routinely on such things as bedsores, catheterization, psychotropic medication, restraints, and falls. They pay close attention to such issues as palliative care to help people end their lives in comfort and dignity, surrounded by family or friends, without aggressive medical intervention.

"We try to help our residents make more appropriate life choices whether they have six weeks or six years left," she said. "Unlike in the past, most people today will die of chronic diseases. Our society's challenge is helping people live with those chronic diseases. In many cases, the nursing home is not a place they will visit and leave. It is their home. So we don't want to send them to hospitals when they get sick. We want to treat them. It is bad for the frail elderly to be sent around to other places. So our role has increased and will continue to do so. The Teaching Nursing Home Program taught everyone the value of high-level, humane care in the nursing home. We're continuing that tradition."

The program's legacy does not rest only in the likes of Debbie Gunter, however. Geraldine Bednash, executive director of the American Association of Colleges of Nursing, said her members had been expressing renewed interest in establishing teaching nursing homes.

"I believe the growing awareness of the need to improve the nursing care dynamics in long-term care settings and the interest in having more meaningful learning opportunities in these settings are coming together to create the potential for some new efforts here," she said. "I am not able to say that anything is in place yet, but we will begin these efforts in earnest."

Meanwhile, even without an organized effort, a few new teaching nursing homes are starting to appear on the horizon. In Lubbock, Texas, for example, Texas Tech University Health Sciences Center has established a $15 million facility with 120 beds, half of them for people needing skilled nursing services and the other half for people with Alzheimer's and other dementia-related illnesses. Students do clinical and research work there. Certified nurse assistants, the core of nursing home staff, are being trained there as well. Social work, law, nursing, pharmacy, and medical students work in an interdisciplinary fashion to develop programs for what they call "healthy aging," said Ana Valdez, associate dean for undergraduates at Texas Tech University Health Sciences Center. She said the original Teaching Nursing Home Program served as the inspiration for the setup.

Finally, the evaluation of the Teaching Nursing Home Program played a role in sharpening the way care of the elderly is evaluated. Peter Shaughnessy of the University of Colorado said that in 1995 the Health Care Financing Administration, responsible for overseeing Medicare and Medicaid, funded a national demonstration project to improve care in fifty-four home health care agencies using an outcome-based quality improvement methodology. In 1999, the Centers for Medicare & Medicaid Services adopted the data set that underpins the methodology for the nation's seven thousand certified home health care agencies and, as of 2003, required its use as the basis for reporting the performance of the nation's certified home health care agencies.[11] As Shaughnessy put it, "It is important to note that the outcome measure system for this quality improvement program has its origins in the outcome measure research done on the Teaching Nursing Home study."

Given that teaching nursing homes were a low-cost, and today only dimly remembered, Foundation pilot project of the 1980s, their legacy, all told, is not a bad one.

## Notes

1. Vladeck, B. *Unloving Care: The Nursing Home Tragedy.* New York: Basic Books, 1980.
2. Aiken, L. H., Mezey, M. D., Lynaugh, J. E., and Buck, C. R. "Teaching Nursing Homes: Prospects for Improving Long Term Care." *Journal of the American Geriatrics Society,* 1976, *33*(3), 96–201.
3. Quotation from "A Perspective of Hope," a 1987 documentary produced by B. Achtenberg, C. Mitchell, and S. Shaw.
4. For a comprehensive look, see Joel, L. A., and Johnson, J. W. "Rutgers—The State University of New Jersey and Bergen Pines County Hospital." In N. R. Small and M. B. Walsh (eds.), *Teaching Nursing Homes: The Nursing Perspective.* Owings Mills, Md.: National Health Publishing, 1988, pp. 211–237.

5. Shaughnessy, P., Kramer, A., Hittle, D., and Steiner, J. "Quality of Care in Teaching Nursing Homes: Findings and Implications." *Health Care Financing Review,* Summer 1995, pp. 55–83.
6. Joel and Johnson (1988).
7. Ibid., pp. 228–229.
8. Quoted by Dexter Hutchins in an unpublished interview for The Robert Wood Johnson Foundation in 2000.
9. Shaughnessy, Kramer, Hittle, and Steiner (1995).
10. Ibid., p. 69.
11. Shaughnessy, P., Crisler, K., and Schlenker, R. "Outcome-Based Quality Improvement in the Information Age." *Home Health Care Management and Practice,* Feb. 1998, pp. 11–18.

# Human Capital Portfolio

# The Robert Wood Johnson Clinical Scholars Program

*Jonathan Showstack, Arlyss Anderson Rothman,*
*Laura C. Leviton, and Lewis G. Sandy*

## Editors' Introduction

Since its earliest days, The Robert Wood Johnson Foundation has recognized the importance of developing leadership capacity in the health sector. Between 1972 and the present, the Foundation has committed nearly $775 million to programs designed to improve the health care workforce. Many of these programs have been the topics of chapters in The Robert Wood Johnson Foundation *Anthology*.[1]

The Clinical Scholars Program, the Foundation's longest-running initiative, is often referred to as its flagship program. Since 1972, the Foundation, through this program, has supported postdoctoral training for young physicians interested in research and leadership careers in health policy.[2] The result is a fraternity of more than nine hundred physicians who have participated in the program and helped to shape the field of health services research.

This chapter examines the Clinical Scholars Program from its inception and builds on a recent evaluation of it conducted by the University of California, San Francisco, or UCSF. It explains why a philanthropy such as The Robert Wood Johnson Foundation would be interested in an expensive, long-term investment like the Clinical Scholars Program and describes how this program has influenced the fields of medicine and health services research over the past thirty-five years. It also raises thoughtful questions about the continued logic of such an initiative in the current health care world.

The chapter was written by Jonathan Showstack, a professor at UCSF, who led the recent evaluation; Arlyss Anderson Rothman, an assistant professor of family health care nursing at UCSF, who participated in the evaluation; Laura Leviton, a senior evaluation officer at The Robert Wood Johnson Foundation; and Lewis Sandy, the Foundation's former executive vice president, who oversaw the Clinical Scholars Program while he was at the Foundation.

1. Isaacs, S. L., Sandy, L. G., and Schroeder, S. A. "Improving the Health Care Workforce: Perspectives from Twenty-Four Years' Experience." In *To Improve Health and Health Care 1997: The Robert Wood Johnson Foundation Anthology.* San Francisco: Jossey-Bass, 1997; Keenan, T. "Support of Nurse Practitioners and Physician Assistants." In *To Improve Health and Health Care 1998–1999: The Robert Wood Johnson Foundation Anthology.* San Francisco: Jossey-Bass, 1998; Frank, R. S. "The Health Policy Fellowships Program." In *To Improve Health and Health Care, Vol. V: The Robert Wood Johnson Foundation Anthology.* San Francisco: Jossey-Bass, 2002; Colby, D. C. "Building Health Policy Research Capacity in the Social Sciences." In *To Improve Health and Health Care, Vol. VI: The Robert Wood Johnson Foundation Anthology.* San Francisco: Jossey-Bass, 2003.
2. The Robert Wood Johnson Foundation took over and modified the program, which had been started by the Carnegie Corporation of New York and the Commonwealth Fund in 1969.

—w— The five senior professors of medicine were an unlikely group to start a revolution. It was the late 1960s, however—a time of social turmoil, idealism, and questioning the status quo. As the professors had lunch together on the final day of a conference on medical education, they were uneasy about the business-as-usual discussions at the meeting. All of them had seen their schools grow rapidly as new research and patient care dollars flowed from the government, yet they shared a concern that all was not right with the way physicians were being educated. Many of their medical students wanted to put action behind their idealism, to spend their careers in policy positions where they could have an impact, not in white coats in a biomedical lab. The professors also recognized that changes in society would have an enormous impact on health and health care over the coming decades and that these changes would require a new type of physician—one who could ask and answer new kinds of questions, understand the changes that were occurring, and have the skills necessary to design, implement, and evaluate new ways of delivering care.

As luck would have it, Margaret Mahoney, a program officer at the Carnegie Corporation of New York, which was sponsoring the conference, was also at the table, and she encouraged them to develop their ideas and send a proposal to her. What resulted from these discussions was the Clinical Scholars Program.

With support from the Carnegie Corporation and the Commonwealth Fund, the Clinical Scholars Program started in 1969 with the funding of five initial sites, each directed by one of the professors of medicine: John Beck at McGill University Faculty of Medicine; Halsted Holman at Stanford University School of Medicine; Julius Krevans at The Johns Hopkins University School of Medicine; Austin Weisberger at Case Western Reserve School of Medicine; and James Wyngaarden at Duke University School of Medicine.

In order to expand and provide long-term support for the Clinical Scholars Program, in 1972 The Robert Wood Johnson Foundation, then a newly established philanthropy, assumed responsibility for the program. The Foundation's new president was David Rogers, a former dean of the school of medicine at Johns Hopkins and someone who was also acutely aware of the issues facing the health care system. The Foundation was interested in identifying and funding new efforts to achieve its goal of improving the health and health care of the American people, and the Clinical Scholars Program seemed like a perfect fit. Both Margaret Mahoney and Terrance Keenan, a program officer at the Commonwealth Fund, had joined The Robert Wood Johnson Foundation staff and would help administer the program, with the name officially changed to the Robert Wood Johnson Clinical Scholars Program. Among other changes that occurred in the early years of sponsorship were the formalization of the application process, the formation of a National Advisory Committee consisting of leaders in medicine and health care, and a new competition for site funding, with some of the original sites not being refunded and new sites added. Beck moved to the University of California, San Francisco, to direct the program initially. Annie Lea Shuster, then a program officer at The Robert Wood Johnson Foundation, assumed responsibility for overseeing the program and continued in this role for over two decades.

## —ᴡ— The Need

Why was a new type of fellowship program needed? Physicians in training can generally become licensed to practice medicine after one year of post–medical school training—their internship year. Beginning in the 1930s, however, residencies extended this training with the goal of certification in a particular specialty. To be eligible for certification, internists, for example, need three years of post–medical school education, which is generally performed at a teaching hospital that is associated with a medical school.

The tremendous increase in medical knowledge in the 1950s and 1960s, and the application of this knowledge through new procedures and technologies, created an incentive to subspecialize, that is, to add several additional years of training after the residency in a particular aspect of care. This type of training is known as a fellowship and can extend training for an additional two years or more. By the late 1960s, for example, it was common for internists to subspecialize in cardiology, gastroenterology, or infectious disease; for pediatricians to subspecialize in neonatology; and for surgeons to subspecialize in orthopedics.

While this trend toward subspecialization was a logical response to a growing knowledge base in medicine, it tended to create physicians whose training was deep but narrow. What kind of physician would retain a broad perspective on health, health care, and medicine in the future? At least in part in reaction to the trend toward subspecialization, family medicine was established as a specialty in the late 1960s to train physicians in a broad set of skills, including care of both adults and children and the ability to perform minor surgery. These family physicians would practice in a wide range of settings and geographic areas. Similarly, in the late 1970s general internal medicine programs were established to train internists to be primary care physicians.

Although subspecialty training produced highly skilled physicians, the five professors of medicine had the foresight to know that the changing health care environment also required physicians with a different type of specialized skills. The next generation of leaders in medicine would need to pose research questions on the organization and financing of health services; on the contribution of medical care to overall population health; and on the relationships between economic, social, and demographic forces on health care, just to name a few areas of inquiry. They would need to work closely with administrators and policymakers to design and implement new systems of care to take advantage of new knowledge and technology and to address the inevitable social, ethical, economic, and legal issues and dilemmas facing American medicine and society.

Heretofore, for a physician who was interested in a career in community or population health, the educational choices were relatively limited—perhaps one or two years at a school of public health or a stint with the Epidemic Intelligence Service of the Centers for Disease Control. No fellowship program, however, provided an integrated educational experience that would give participants the knowledge and skills in population health, epidemiology, research methods, health care organization, economics, and health policy that would be needed by future leaders in medicine.

The Clinical Scholars Program was designed to produce scholarly physician-leaders with the understanding and the skills necessary to have a major influence on health care policy, to help create and build the relatively new field of health services research, and to thrive in academic medicine. It was conceived as, and continues to be, a two-year fellowship for physicians who have completed their initial clinical training, with most Clinical Scholars joining the program directly after residency.

Over the past thirty years, the program's goals have remained relatively constant while the program itself has gone through expansions and contractions, the eligibility criteria for appointment as a Clinical Scholar have broadened, and program sites have changed. The methods used at each of the sites have generally included seminars in health policy, epidemiology, biostatistics, research methods, and economics, and an applied research experience. Over time, sites have tended to develop unique areas of emphasis. Yale, for example, focused on clinical epidemiology; UCLA, on health services research; and the joint University of California, San Francisco–Stanford site, on chronic illness. This specialization was a useful way to attract scholars with particular interests and to use the sometimes unique resources available at each site. Scholars are expected to design and conduct a relevant research project during their fellowship, as well as to continue caring for patients (to maintain their clinical skills and to ground their academic experience in the reality of today's health care system).

## —᠁— The Clinical Scholars

To date, the program has had over nine hundred graduates. Most Clinical Scholars begin their careers within academic medicine, undertaking policy-relevant health services research. Over time, many have become leaders in health policy, health services research, clinical epidemiology, and population health. Graduates have become directors of major federal, state, and local health agencies and departments, chairs of departments in medical schools, chief executive officers of hospitals, influential researchers in the fields of health services and health economics, and foundation executives (including the current president and the former executive vice president of The Robert Wood Johnson Foundation). Among the program's alumni, there are approximately 150 full professors and over twenty

**Table 5.1** Clinical Scholar Program Sites

| Program Site | Dates of Program* |
|---|---|
| Case Western Reserve University | 1969†–1977 |
| Columbia University | 1975–1979 |
| Duke University | 1969†–1975 |
| George Washington University | 1975–1979 |
| Johns Hopkins University | 1969†–1978, 1995–2003 |
| McGill University | 1970†–1981 |
| University of California, Los Angeles | 1975–2003 |
| UCSF-Stanford‡ | 1970†–1996 |
| University of Chicago | 1995–2003 |
| University of Michigan | 1995–2003 |
| University of North Carolina | 1973–2003 |
| University of Pennsylvania | 1973–2003 |
| University of Washington | 1975–2003 |
| Yale University | 1974–2003 |

*Dates when scholars were in residence at program site.
†These programs were supported by the Carnegie Corporation and the Commonwealth Fund until 1972, at which time The Robert Wood Johnson Foundation assumed responsibility for the program.
‡University of California, San Francisco–Stanford University joint program.
*Source:* Showstack, J., Anderson Rothman, A., and Greene, N. *Survey of the Market for the Clinical Scholars Program: Final Report Submitted to The Robert Wood Johnson Foundation.* (Unpublished). 2002.

current chairs of medical school departments. More than thirty former Clinical Scholars have been elected to the Institute of Medicine of the National Academy of Sciences. Although many Clinical Scholars choose to work within their training institutions after completion of the program, graduates have dispersed geographically throughout the United States and are found in every state.

Participants in the Clinical Scholars Program have come from many areas of medicine. The majority were trained in internal medicine, with pediatricians the next largest group, followed by those trained in family medicine, psychiatry, obstetrics and gynecology, preventive medicine, emergency medicine, surgery, occupational medicine, community medicine, radiology, and public health. Although the majority of Clinical Scholars have been men, in recent years there have been approximately equal numbers of men and women in the program.

## —⟋⟍— Program Impact

The Clinical Scholars Program has had an impact on health policy and health services research; on the sites where the program has been implemented; on other fellowships; and on the Foundation itself.

### *Impact on Health Policy and Health Services Research*

By making a long-term commitment to training hundreds of clinicians in health services and health policy research, the program helped legitimize and institutionalize these fields within academic medicine. In contrast to the early years of the program, when health services research was a foreign concept in academic medicine, virtually all research-intensive medical schools now have active health services research programs. The National Institutes of Health, the leading funder of medical research, has added this kind of research to its agenda, and physicians, along with social scientists, are now leaders in the field.

Clinical Scholars have been involved in some of the most influential studies in health policy over the past thirty years. For example, former Clinical Scholar Robert Brook played a major role in the RAND Health Insurance Experiment, a landmark study to determine whether increased copayments for patients would affect their utilization of medical services. In the late 1970s and early 1980s, former Clinical Scholars published studies demonstrating wide variation in the use of medical procedures in different regions of the United States and a resulting overuse, underuse, and misuse of therapies. These studies led to an increased focus on clinical practice guidelines, for which the expertise of Clinical Scholars and other physician-researchers was critical.

Studies such as these and the growing influence of health services researchers in academia catalyzed the development of a national infrastructure for health policy and health services research, which, in turn, created new opportunities for Clinical Scholars. In 1989, Congress created the Agency for Health Care Policy and Research to fund outcomes research and develop practice guidelines. The agency (now the Agency for Healthcare Research and Quality) has provided funding to physician health services researchers and wielded a considerable influence on efforts to improve the quality of medical care. In 1997, former Clinical Scholar John Eisenberg became the agency's director (a position he held until his death in 2002), and the program's graduates have held high-level positions in the Centers for Medicare & Medicaid Services (formerly the Health Care Financing Administration).

### Impact on the Program Sites and on Other Fellowships

In supporting institutions as training sites for the Clinical Scholars Program, the Foundation offered more than just stipend support for those selected as Clinical Scholars; it also provided funding for the program's site director and core faculty members at the sites, essentially building a small academic unit. In a 1992 evaluation of the program, Harvard University health economist Rashi Fein and then-president of New York City's Mt. Sinai Medical Center John Rowe spoke with deans and department chairs of medical schools participating in the Clinical Scholars Program, all of whom agreed that the program had changed the intellectual climate of their institutions for the better. It had, they said, increased the interest in and respect for epidemiological research and led to more health services research, even outside the program's traditional base of departments of medicine and pediatrics. Additionally, the subject matter of the Clinical Scholars Program had influenced the schools' curricula. Finally, the host institutions consistently showed an interest in keeping Clinical Scholars on their faculty after they completed the program.

The unpublished report by Fein and Rowe noted that academic leaders at the University of Pennsylvania credited the Clinical Scholars Program with helping to foster an academic program in geriatrics; that Clinical Scholars and the program's faculty at Yale had supported development of multidisciplinary geriatric research; and that the program's faculty at the University of Washington had developed courses for the Clinical Scholars that were later added to the general curriculum.

In addition, the Fein and Rowe report pointed out that a substantial number of training opportunities could be said to derive in part from the Clinical Scholars Program. These included the National Research Service

Awards and the Physician Scientist Awards, both given by the National Institutes of Health or its component institutes. In addition, at least thirteen institutions had created programs similar to Clinical Scholars with other funding.

### *Impact on The Robert Wood Johnson Foundation*

The Clinical Scholars Program has influenced the Foundation's grantmaking in a number of ways. First, the Foundation's leadership and staff regularly call upon former Clinical Scholars as experts, consultants, or program directors. Second, the research and policy interests of Clinical Scholars have helped inform the Foundation of important, emerging areas. For example, in the mid-1980s former Clinical Scholars William Knaus and Joanne Lynn became interested in improving end-of-life care. This interest led the Foundation to fund SUPPORT, a landmark study on improving care and respecting the wishes of dying patients and, later, to a major initiative to improve the quality of care toward the end of people's lives.

Third, the program has had an impact on the Foundation's grantmaking strategies. Because the Clinical Scholars is widely regarded within the Foundation as successful, it has served as the model, to one degree or another, for other Foundation fellowship programs. For example, the proposal for the Scholars in Health Policy Research Program, which is designed to attract top-tier economists, political scientists, and sociologists into health policy research, pointed out that, as in the case of Clinical Scholars, the "prestige factor" would help increase attention to health policy research among these disciplines. To achieve this level of prestige, the program is located at highly rated universities and aims at attracting the very best young Ph.D.'s into health policy research. The program aspires, as well, to have the same kind of positive effects on faculty, curriculum, and the field of health services research as the Clinical Scholars Program has had.

More generally, the widely perceived success of the Clinical Scholars Program provides a justification for the Foundation's investments in human capital. Identifying, supporting, and nurturing leaders is believed to be an effective long-term philanthropic strategy, although one whose payoff is difficult to measure and may not be readily discernable for a decade or more. Recognizing this, The Robert Wood Johnson Foundation recently created a team and grantmaking portfolio dedicated to supporting the development of human capital.

## —ɯ— Clinical Scholars in a Changing Marketplace

Medicine and American society have undergone major changes since the program's birth in the late 1960s. After enjoying almost unfettered growth in the 1960s and 1970s, academic medicine began to face the financial challenges of a changing marketplace. From the 1970s through the early 1990s, the health care system grew with seemingly little restraint. Academic health centers were among the chief beneficiaries of this growth. Jobs in health care were plentiful; there were great career opportunities in health care administration and policy; faculties in medical schools were expanding rapidly; and funding for research was readily available. Times were good for the graduates of the Clinical Scholars Program.

In their 1992 evaluation, Fein and Rowe concluded that the program was successful, praising it as "a national treasure."[1] They recommended that it be continued, with some adjustments, such as changing the locations of program sites and holding new competitions for them. These recommendations were adopted.

At about the time that Fein and Rowe assessed the program, great changes in health care and medical education were beginning to appear. These were to have a significant impact on the program.

First, resources did not flow into medical care as rapidly as before, and increased competition and lower reimbursement began eating into the revenues of academic health centers. By the late 1990s, there were disquieting signs that the graduates of the Clinical Scholars Program were not finding the job market as expansive as did their predecessors.

Second, perhaps because of the success of the Clinical Scholars Program, a number of new fellowship programs had been developed in the late 1980s and 1990s that competed directly for the same pool of applicants as the Clinical Scholars Program. These included the National Research Service Awards, the Veterans Administration National Quality Scholars Fellowship Program, career development awards from the National Institutes of Health and Agency for Healthcare Research and Quality, and general internal medicine fellowships. Many of these competing fellowship programs included training that was similar to that received by the Clinical Scholars and were both easier to get into and shorter in length.

Third, the 1990s saw significant demographic and financial changes in health care. The most important of these changes were the increased number of women in medical schools (the entering medical school class in the late 1980s was about one-third female; today it is about half), the ebb and flow of interest in primary care, and the increasing debt incurred by medical students due to rising tuition costs. Women's career paths and lifestyle choices tend to differ from men's, largely because of childbearing and family commitments. This makes spending additional years in fellowship programs a less desirable option for many women. A decreased interest in primary care—which occurred in the late 1990s—diminished the pool of physicians of the kind who normally apply to become Clinical Scholars. In addition, the financial burden of medical school may have caused some young physicians to reject fellowship training in favor of taking jobs directly after residency training and paying off their debts.

As the renewal of the Clinical Scholars Program approached in the late 1990s, the Foundation felt that it was time to reassess the program. To inform discussions about the future directions of the Clinical Scholars Program, the Foundation asked a team at UCSF to examine whether the Clinical Scholars Program was still a popular choice among potential applicants and whether the career progression of Clinical Scholars was as rapid as in past years.

To assess the attractiveness of the program, UCSF conducted a survey of the career choices of those who traditionally consider applying to the Clinical Scholars Program—second- and third-year primary care residents in family medicine, general internal medicine, and pediatrics. In a second part of the study, all current and former Clinical Scholars were asked to complete a survey about their experience in the Clinical Scholars Program, their career paths, and current positions. In this way, the career paths of Clinical Scholars who graduated in different periods could be compared. In all, over six hundred residents responded to the first survey, and nearly half of the over nine hundred current and former scholars responded.

## Future Scholars: The Career Goals of Today's Primary Care Residents

The primary career goal of the majority of the residents who responded to the survey was clinical practice. General internal medicine and pediatric residents were three times as likely as family medicine residents to indicate academia as a possible job option.

The main reasons that the residents were considering fellowship training were to specialize, to increase their knowledge, and as a route into academics. As shown in Figure 5.1, two-thirds of internal medicine residents, about one-half of pediatrics residents, and about a third of family medicine residents indicated an interest in fellowship training. Only one in ten said that they would apply to a nonsubspecialty fellowship, and only a handful mentioned the Clinical Scholars Program as a possibility.

The national reputation of a fellowship program, its placement of graduates, and its research reputation were rated as important by most residents, with family medicine residents placing less emphasis on research

**Figure 5.1**  Residents Are Primarily Interested in Subspecialty Fellowships

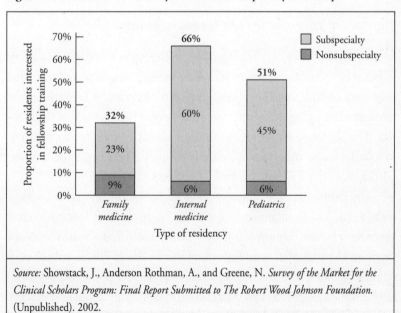

Source: Showstack, J., Anderson Rothman, A., and Greene, N. *Survey of the Market for the Clinical Scholars Program: Final Report Submitted to The Robert Wood Johnson Foundation.* (Unpublished). 2002.

reputation. The most highly rated attribute for a fellowship program was the availability of a mentor, followed by the quality of the program as evidenced by its national reputation and the recommendation of an adviser. Other important considerations in choosing a program included the location of the fellowship, suitability for a partner, and the availability of research support and protected time.

Most primary care residents who were considering further training intended to apply to a subspecialty fellowship, with only a small portion (7 percent) considering applying to a nonsubspecialty program. Sponsorship by The Robert Wood Johnson Foundation was rated as important by relatively few (13 percent) of the residents.

These results suggest that the Clinical Scholars Program may not be as competitive and attractive a choice for primary care residents as it was in earlier years.

In addition, the results emphasize the importance of mentoring and the overall quality of the program. The data provided important lessons for the program going forward. In particular, the mentoring component, always a strong element, would receive even greater emphasis in the years ahead.

### *The Career Trajectories of Clinical Scholars*

Almost half of the current and former scholars replied to the survey. Most Clinical Scholars identified an academic career as a goal at the time that they were considering the Clinical Scholars Program, with only a small number identifying other options, such as government or clinical practice. The perceived quality of the Clinical Scholars Program was the most influential factor in scholars' decisions to apply to the program; this was particularly true for more recent Clinical Scholars.

The debt burden of recent medical school graduates and changes in social needs had an increasingly important effect on the fellowship choices made by scholars. As shown in Figure 5.2, financial constraints were not mentioned by scholars who had graduated in the 1970s, but these constraints had an increasing impact over time. Partner preferences, including family, employment, and other issues, affected only about one in seven scholars in the 1970s, but over a third of them in the 1990s.

**Figure 5.2** Personal and Financial Issues Have Increased in Importance

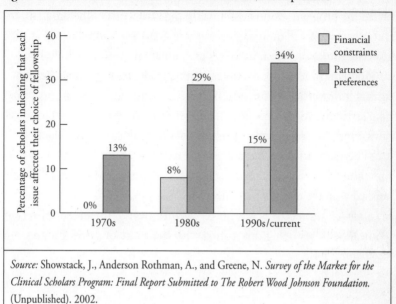

*Source:* Showstack, J., Anderson Rothman, A., and Greene, N. *Survey of the Market for the Clinical Scholars Program: Final Report Submitted to The Robert Wood Johnson Foundation.* (Unpublished). 2002.

The vast majority of scholars (87 percent overall) said that they had gained what they had hoped for from the program, with one in four saying that they achieved the maximum benefit from the program that they thought possible. There was, however, a small but important increase in the proportion of scholars in the 1990s cohort who said that they had gained only part or none of what they had hoped. Additional gains that had not been anticipated included networking, program content, career development, and mentoring. A small proportion, but increasing over time, said that there was a need for better mentoring, and the need for an additional (third) year was mentioned by a number of more recent Clinical Scholars.

In the program's first two decades, most graduates of the Clinical Scholars Program were able to obtain the type of job that they desired. During the 1990s, however, a decreasing proportion of scholars said that they were able to obtain the type of job that they wanted. Compared with Clinical Scholars in earlier years, approximately twice as many scholars in the 1990s found their job searches to be more difficult than expected.

The first job for three out of four Clinical Scholars after they completed the program was in academia. In the early years of the program, career progression was quite rapid; over one-quarter advanced to the level of associate professor within five years of graduation from the Clinical Scholars Program. In recent years, the program's graduates began their academic careers in lower-level positions (lectureship and similar positions rather than assistant professor positions, and fewer scholars in tenure-track positions), and their rate of advancement slowed significantly (see Figure 5.3).

The perception of the program's graduates about their careers mirrors these objective data. Most scholars who graduated in the 1970s are satisfied with the rate at which their career has progressed. This has changed dramatically in recent years, however, with nearly 40 percent of recent Clinical Scholars being dissatisfied with their rate of career progression (see Figure 5.4).

**Figure 5.3** Academic Advancement Has Slowed for Recent Scholars

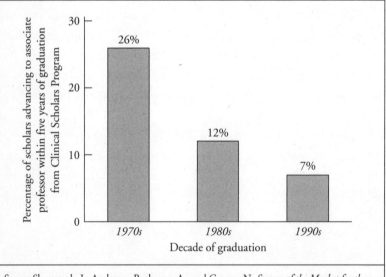

Source: Showstack, J., Anderson Rothman, A., and Greene, N. *Survey of the Market for the Clinical Scholars Program: Final Report Submitted to The Robert Wood Johnson Foundation.* (Unpublished). 2002.

**Figure 5.4** Recent Scholars Are Less Satisfied with Their Rate of Career Advancement

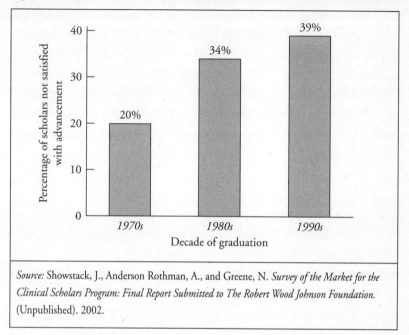

*Source:* Showstack, J., Anderson Rothman, A., and Greene, N. *Survey of the Market for the Clinical Scholars Program: Final Report Submitted to The Robert Wood Johnson Foundation.* (Unpublished). 2002.

## *Implications for the Clinical Scholars Program*

The surveys of primary care residents and current and former Clinical Scholars suggest a more competitive environment for fellowship programs as they try to attract applicants and for graduates of the Clinical Scholars Program as they enter the job market. The high proportion of primary care residents, especially of general internal medicine residents, who intend to subspecialize is sobering. The trend toward subspecialization by primary care residents and their general lack of awareness of The Robert Wood Johnson Foundation or the Clinical Scholars Program suggest that the potential pool of applicants for the program has declined and may continue to decline over time. Or it may well be that the traditional sources of Clinical Scholars will become a smaller proportion of the applicant pool, with more Clinical Scholars applying from medical and surgical specialties.

There has been a clear and significant increase in the challenges faced by recent scholars in their ability to get the jobs that they want and in their overall career advancement. In a sense, the very success of the Clinical Scholars Program may be the indirect cause of some of the difficulties faced by recent graduates of the program, with increasing competition from graduates of similar fellowships for a relatively limited number of jobs. Perhaps the most important finding from the survey of current and former Clinical Scholars, however, was their overwhelming endorsement of the program.

## —ɯ— The Future

With its emphasis on health services research and health care policy, the Clinical Scholars Program was unique among fellowship programs available in the 1970s and early 1980s. The program has been, and continues to be, impressive. Changes in medical care and in society as a whole present new challenges as the program enters its fourth decade.

In 2002, as The Robert Wood Johnson Foundation considered the future of the program, the record of its graduates, and the changing environment in medicine and health care, a number of options emerged. One option was to "declare victory" and devote resources to other programs and challenges. Another option was to take an "if it isn't broken, don't fix it" position and continue the program with minor changes. What the Foundation ultimately decided, however, was to revamp the Clinical Scholars Program in a way that would continue its aims, while structuring it for the twenty-first-century environment in academic medicine and society. It did this in five ways.

First, as it had done previously, the Foundation launched a new, national competition for sites; these new sites would enroll Clinical Scholars beginning in 2005. Second, it adjusted the program to give greater structure to the core curriculum, more explicit productivity expectations, and more emphasis on primary data collection and community-based research. Third, it added an optional third year (available by application to the program). Fourth, it created a whole new program for early career development to provide support for recent graduates of the Clinical Scholars

Program, as well as those from other similar fellowship programs. This new program, approved by the Foundation's trustees in 2002, will provide new opportunities for mentoring and networking for current and former Clinical Scholars. Finally, it shifted the program's leadership and placed it under the direction of Iris Litt, the Marron and Mary Elizabeth Kendrick Professor of Pediatrics at Stanford University.

While it may take a decade or more to determine the impact of the program changes, the Foundation believes that investing in talented young people continues to be a good bet and a winning philanthropic strategy. As was the case in the late 1960s, when the five senior professors of medicine saw a need for a new type of fellowship program, profound changes continue to occur in society and in the medical care system that require new and innovative ways to prevent illness and to care for those who become ill. Outstanding clinicians, trained to ask and answer important questions, well versed in the policy process, and with an inclination toward action that improves health and health care, will continue to make a positive impact.

## Note

1. Fein, R., and Rowe, J. *A Review of the Clinical Scholars Program.* (Unpublished). Report prepared for The Robert Wood Johnson Foundation, 1992.

# The Robert Wood Johnson Foundation's Commitment to Increasing Minorities in the Health Professions

*Jane Isaacs Lowe and Constance M. Pechura*

## Editors' Introduction

This chapter reviews the strategies The Robert Wood Johnson Foundation has pursued to increase the number of minority physicians, nurses, and other health care providers. This has been a priority for the Foundation since it emerged as a national philanthropy in 1972. Among its first grantees, in fact, was a medical school scholarship fund for minorities, women, and inhabitants of rural areas.

The motivation behind the Foundation's interest in minority health practitioners has always been to improve access to and the quality of care for minority patients. Research indicates that minority practitioners are more likely than

The authors of this chapter are indebted to the following people who provided valuable insight and information: Robert Blendon, Joel Cantor, James Gavin, Ruby Hearn, James Ingram, Terrance Keenan, and Margaret Mahoney. Special thanks to Ayorkor Gaba for her research assistance and to Anita Calicchio and Toni Scratchard for their administrative assistance.

majority practitioners to work in low-income communities and to have practices that serve larger proportions of minority populations. Studies on sociocultural barriers to health care services show that members of minorities are more likely to seek services from, and follow the medical advice of, minority providers. This is particularly true in the case of non-English-speaking patients.

The authors of the chapter—Foundation senior program officers Jane Isaacs Lowe and Constance M. Pechura—have been active in shaping the Foundation's recent strategies in the areas of minority medical workforce and, more generally, human capital. Lowe heads the Foundation's team on services for vulnerable populations and monitors a number of the programs directed at improving the minority health care workforce. Pechura leads a team overseeing the Foundation's investments to improve human capital in the health sector.

The Foundation's programs to encourage minorities to enter the health care workforce cannot be understood apart from the greater social policy debate about race in the United States. Even though the programs funded by the Foundation cannot reasonably be characterized as affirmative action, they must be seen within the context of this divisive issue. In the chapter, Lowe and Pechura examine the 2003 Supreme Court affirmative action decisions and their potential effect on programs to increase minorities in the health care workforce.

—⚇— **I**n the 1960s, major social upheavals had begun to bring permanent and fundamental change to the United States, and the country became galvanized to right the wrongs of the past and take responsibility for its most vulnerable citizens. The civil rights movement reached a pinnacle at this time as freedom rides, boycotts, and civil unrest led to major political actions. The Civil Rights Act, the War on Poverty, and Medicaid and Medicare were all products of the sixties. They were part of a general trend to increase the role of the federal government and federal law in effecting social change. In response to a predicted shortage of health care professionals, Congress passed the Health Professions Educational Assistance Act of 1963. The law provided, for the first time, government-sponsored financial aid for the health professions and increased the number of medical schools. Twenty-five new medical schools were established between 1963 and 1975, and the number of medical students rose from about thirty-three thousand to fifty-six thousand.

The philanthropic sector had been working on the problem of underrepresented minorities in medicine even before the 1960s.[1] Some well-established foundations, including the Ford Foundation, the Carnegie Corporation, and the Rockefeller Brothers Fund, were supporting black colleges and the United Negro College Fund. The National Medical Fellowships, which had been established in 1946 as Provident Medical Associates, provided scholarships for African American, Hispanic, and Native American medical students. The Julius Rosenwald Fund, the Field Foundation, the Commonwealth Fund, and the Alfred P. Sloan Foundation provided support to it as far back as the 1940s.[2]

With the Civil Rights Act in place, other philanthropies became more actively involved. The Josiah Macy, Jr. Foundation, for example, began, in 1966, to fund medical schools to establish formal offices that would address minority recruitment. The Association of American Medical Colleges, or AAMC, embraced these efforts and took an early lead in the effort to increase minorities in medicine. By 1971, the U.S. Office of Economic Opportunity, through the AAMC, was providing funds to increase minority participation in medicine under the Special Health Career Opportunity Grant Program.

So the stage seemed to be set to increase access to health care for all Americans and to open the doors of health professions to minorities and those previously unable to afford higher education. These two thrusts were thought to be intricately connected, since many people in the field believed that blacks and other minority health professionals would be more likely to practice in poor, minority areas. Yet the percentage of minorities entering the health professions was far below their representation in the total population. In 1970, for example, only 2.4 percent of the nation's medical students and 5.9 percent of its medical professionals were minorities, even though minorities constituted 16 percent of the general population.[3]

## —⟋⟍— Early Programming at The Robert Wood Johnson Foundation

The Robert Wood Johnson Foundation was born into this social environment in 1972, with a mandate to improve the health and health care of all Americans. The Foundation's board of trustees established, as one of its first priorities, increasing access to medical care. Reflecting this priority, the Foundation took three early steps. First, in 1972, it funded a scholarship and loan program for women, minorities, and people from rural areas who wanted to attend medical or dental school (awarding the money quickly also helped it to satisfy the requirements of the Internal Revenue Service).[4] This was supplemented in 1973 by grants to National Medical Fellowships, Inc., to enhance its scholarship fund for minority students. Second, the Foundation made a grant to the College of Medicine and Dentistry of New Jersey for a summer enrichment program for minority students entering medical or dental school. The third step was to provide institutional support to Meharry Medical College, which, at the time, was one of only two four-year medical schools specifically training African Americans. Meharry was training about 40 percent of all black physicians and dentists, and the other school, at Howard University, had substantial, albeit insufficient, federal support. Both the Charles R. Drew Postgraduate School (now the Charles R. Drew University of Medicine and Science) and Morehouse College offered only the first two years of medical school curricula.

Although many members of the staff and the board may have been personally committed to civil rights throughout the 1970s and the early 1980s, the justification for the Foundation's minority programs was strictly a health one—to increase access to care among underserved populations. Grants to enable more minorities (and women and those living in rural areas) to become physicians and dentists were justified by the belief that these groups would be more likely to practice primary care in inner cities and rural areas. Later studies have provided evidence to support this belief.

The student financial aid programs that began in the early 1970s were frequently adjusted, and they resulted in a variety of funding mechanisms. These included grants to individual medical and dental schools for minority student financial aid, continued support to the National Medical Fellowships program (which, over the years, amounted to more than $10 million), and a guaranteed student loan program.

Within The Robert Wood Johnson Foundation, the early work to increase minority representation in medicine and dentistry provided tangible evidence of the Foundation's commitment to increasing access to care. It also formed part of a broader strategy to improve the quality and balance of the health care workforce, as exemplified by initiatives such as the Clinical Scholars Program and the Health Policy Fellowships Program.[5]

Outside the Foundation, the admission of minorities to medical schools was affected by the controversy over affirmative action programs. These were hotly debated and challenged in the courts. Medical school admissions policies came under direct attack in the mid-1970s with the lawsuit of Allan Bakke against the Regents of the University of California, which was decided by the U.S. Supreme Court in 1978. A deeply divided Court struck down the medical school's admissions system, which reserved a certain number of seats for minorities. Justice Lewis Powell, who cast the deciding vote, concluded in his opinion that race, among other factors, could be used as a plus factor in admissions decisions *if* racial diversity supported the educational mission of the school.

Although the Bakke case appeared to provide support for affirmative steps in admissions policies as long as the steps did not involve quotas or set-asides, the ambiguities in the Court's fragmented decision increased the wariness of medical schools in employing affirmative action policies. This wariness decreased in the 1980s because few other court challenges to admissions policies were attempted, and none of them were successful.

In addition to the legal concerns, the high cost of medical and dental education impeded minority enrollment in medical schools, raising the question of whether financial aid was sufficient to attract minority students, whose financial positions were often weak to begin with.

## —⟋⟍— The 1980s and a Change in Focus

At its July 1980 board meeting, The Robert Wood Johnson Foundation's board of trustees charged the staff with examining four options for increasing the number of minority students attending medical school:

1. Creating a national organization to spur interest among minority college students in applying to medical school

2. Supporting programs of intense preparation during college for minority students

3. Continuing support for Meharry Medical College

4. Continuing the Foundation's participation in medical student loan and scholarship programs

By July 1981, the staff had examined some of these options and was considering a number of new approaches. But about that time outside events caused it to reconsider the wisdom of funding new minority programs. First, the federal government threatened to stop funding college student enrichment programs such as the Health Careers Opportunity Program. Second, the government threatened to reduce financial aid for students, even as the cost of a medical education was rising. Third, and most important, the Graduate Medical Education National Advisory Committee issued an influential report that predicted a surplus of 70,000 physicians by 1990 and 145,000 by 2000, and recommended cutting back medical school enrollment. These events led the Foundation to delay authorizing new minority programs in favor of renewing existing ones on a case-by-case basis.

The first case was that of Meharry Medical College, which at the time was beset with fiscal, management, and staffing problems. At its July 1981 meeting, the board considered a staff report examining whether the Foundation should continue its support of Meharry—the nation's largest single educator of black physicians and dentists, a very high percentage of whom practiced in poor, underserved areas and in the rural South. There were potential partners to help The Robert Wood Johnson Foundation: Congress was considering a $4 million to $6 million appropriation of annual special assistance to support Meharry; a national committee of prominent business leaders had taken on the job of leading a major capital campaign; and other foundations (including the Charles Stewart Mott Foundation, the John D. and Catherine T. MacArthur Foundation, and the Commonwealth Fund) had contributed funds to support Meharry's reorganization. The board decided to continue funding Meharry. With the Foundation's support and that of the federal government, members of the business community, and other foundations, Meharry survived.

In March 1982, the Educational Testing Service completed an analysis of the assumptions underlying Robert Wood Johnson Foundation–supported programs aimed at increasing the pool of minorities applying to medical school and improving the performance of minority medical students.[6] The analysis found that minority students did less well than whites on the Medical College Admissions Test, or MCAT, and that the number of qualified African American applicants to medical schools had actually decreased. In 1975, African Americans represented 7.5 percent of the students entering medical school, but that percentage dropped to 6.5 percent by 1980. The decline was due, in part, to increased opportunities for minority candidates in other professional fields, such as engineering and law.[7] The analysis concluded that minority students needed to be better prepared to qualify for, and succeed in, medical school.

Using the results of this study, the Foundation's minority medical education programs began to emerge in 1982. Initially, the Foundation funded three relatively small projects. The first supported the Charles R. Drew Postgraduate School and the Los Angeles Unified School District in building a magnet school to attract minority high school students to the health professions. The second funded a University of Southern California consortium that provided tutorial services to disadvantaged and minority medical school applicants. The third assisted the National Fund for Medical Education in continuing its summer remedial programs for incoming minority medical students.

These experiments in enhancing the skills of minority high school and college students were to lead to a major initiative, but even before that occurred, the Foundation's attention turned to a parallel concern: the role of medical school faculty in the recruitment and retention of minority medical students. A 1978 AAMC task force report on minorities in medicine had called for an increase in the number of minority medical faculty members. The report had made it clear that a major barrier to success for minority students was the scarcity of faculty who "looked like them" or were likely to have come from similar backgrounds. According to the AAMC report, in the 1971–72 academic year there were only 334 African Americans with M.D.'s on medical school faculties, compared with 17,376 whites. That is, African Americans constituted less than 2 percent of the nation's medical school faculty. Four years later, in the 1975–76 academic year, African Americans still constituted less than 2 percent of the nation's medical school faculty members.

The Robert Wood Johnson Foundation's response to this situation was the Minority Medical Faculty Development Program, authorized in 1983. Since success in research was critical to an academic career, the program provided funds for young minority faculty members to spend 70 percent of their time pursuing their research interests. It gave the fellows' institutions money to cover salary, partial research costs over a four-year period, and mentors to help guide the young faculty members in their research efforts. For an applicant to be successful, the choice of a mentor was as important as the project proposed. The active involvement of the program's National Advisory Committee members with each fellow strengthened the mentoring process. A 1995 evaluation of the Minority Medical Faculty Development Program confirmed that the mentoring component was of exceptional importance.[8]

To date, the Minority Medical Faculty Development Program has supported more than two hundred junior minority faculty members. Over 80 percent have remained in academic medicine, and many have become leaders in their fields.[9] Some of its graduates now sit on the National Advisory Committee and have become mentors themselves. Since 1983 the Foundation has invested nearly $80 million in this program.

Once the faculty development program was launched, the Foundation refocused its attention on minority college students. Informal assessments of the previously funded small enrichment programs indicated that they needed to be more structured. In 1987, to provide minority college students with a rigorous academic enrichment on a larger scale, the Foundation established the Minority Medical Education Program. It was set up as a six-week summer residential program for minority students to increase their knowledge and skills, thereby increasing their chance of being accepted into medical school. Funds to the four initial sites supported a standard residential enrichment program, student stipends, and travel costs. Each site offered a structured and multicomponent program, including advanced science and math courses; analytical, writing, test-taking, and oral presentation skills; admissions testing review; application process tutoring; mentoring; and an introduction to clinical practice.

An evaluation of the Minority Medical Education Program found that compared with nonparticipants, significantly higher percentages of the program's participants were accepted into medical schools.[10] Between 1989 and 2001 approximately ten thousand students participated in the Minority Medical Education Program. Nearly all of them have graduated from college, though some are still in school. Of the program participants who already have graduated from college, approximately 49 percent have applied to medical school, and 63 percent of those have been accepted. Those who have completed medical school are represented in all fields of medicine. Since 1987, this program has grown from four to twelve sites, with approximately 1,300 students participating each summer, drawn from colleges and universities across the United States.

Moreover, the model is now widely utilized. By the end of the 1980s, more than a third of the nation's medical schools were sponsoring some type of academic enrichment program for premedical students and students at the postbaccalaureate level, and many were placing high school students in laboratories during the summer.[11] In addition, the Bureau of Health Professions of the U.S. Department of Health and Human Services, through its Health Careers Opportunities Program and Centers of Excellence, continued to provide support to health professions schools for minority students. The Howard Hughes Medical Institute and the National Institutes of Health were funding research opportunities for college students. The Josiah Macy, Jr. Foundation and the Henry J. Kaiser Family Foundation supported magnet high schools that emphasized health and science, as well as after-school and summer programs that provided academic enrichment, counseling, and information about careers in medicine.

Yet, although the numbers have risen, the percentage of minority physicians was still substantially lower than their representation in the general population. A 1987 Special Report on the Foundation's minority medical training programs suggested that after nearly twenty years, these programs did not reach sufficiently large numbers of students and did not address a significant cause of minority underrepresentation—educational disparities in public school education.[12]

## —ᴍ— The 1990s and the Expansion of the Pipeline

In response to growing evidence documenting a leveling in the number of minority medical students, the AAMC designed a program to address inequities in math and science education, particularly in secondary school. Lack of math and science knowledge was seen as the main obstacle to increasing minority admissions to medical school. At the 1991 annual meeting of the AAMC, Robert Petersdorf, the organization's president, challenged medical schools to enroll three thousand underrepresented minority students by the year 2000.[13] Project 3000 by 2000 was launched in 1991 with a Science Education Partnership Award from the National Institutes of Health. This highly promoted initiative encouraged medical schools to increase the size and the quality of underrepresented minority applicants by forming partnerships with elementary and secondary schools, colleges, and community groups.

In 1994, building on the work of the AAMC, The Robert Wood Johnson Foundation developed the Health Professions Partnership Initiative as a way to support the efforts of academic medical centers engaged in Project 3000 by 2000. The aim was to help medical schools and other health professions schools build partnerships with K–12 school systems, colleges, and the communities to improve the quality of math and science teaching and increase students' interest in health careers.

The W. K. Kellogg Foundation and The Robert Wood Johnson Foundation collaborated in this program. The two foundations funded a total of twenty-six new partnerships between 1996 and 2000, including five targeted to increasing underrepresented minorities interested in public health. The lead agency was either a medical or other health professions school; partners were public schools, community agencies, or, in some cases, universities. Each site received $70,000 a year for five years, and all the partners were expected to contribute their own resources toward the program.

The types of activities undertaken by the partnerships varied from academic enrichment programs (tutoring, summer intensive science programs, and instruction in general academic skills) to programs aimed at enhancing schools and teaching (curriculum development, teacher training, and new resources for math and science education).

At the end of the 1990s, the Foundation continued to support the Minority Medical Education Program and the Minority Medical Faculty Development Program. The field is currently emphasizing kindergarten through grade 12 and college pipeline programs to prepare students for careers in medicine and in health services more broadly.[14] Private philanthropic organizations, such as the Howard Hughes Medical Institute and the Josiah Macy, Jr. Foundation, and the federal government, through programs offered by the Bureau of Health Professions, the National Institutes of Health, and the National Science Foundation, provide grants for science and math curriculum reform at the public school level, and enrichment and research programs for high school, college, and medical school students.

## —ᴡᴡ— Observations

1. *First and foremost, expanding the numbers of minority students who are prepared for college and graduate health professions schools remains a high priority.*

The pipeline theoretically begins in elementary school and then flows to junior high, to high school, to college, to graduate education (medical school, nursing), to careers and career advancement. If the problem were in fact that simple, well defined, and linear, it would have been solved decades ago. Instead, the educational systems are failing large numbers of children early on, resulting in a pipeline with large leaks. It is no secret that there are tremendous racial and ethnic disparities in education. Achievement gaps between minority and majority students begin in kindergarten and widen in elementary school. Curriculum tracking begins in middle school, formalizing the gap. This achievement gap has been documented not only in poor inner city schools but also in more affluent suburban schools.[15]

The challenge is to design programs that help to promote high academic achievement and reduce the numbers of students who leave secondary education underprepared. Public school reform, driven at both the state and federal levels, offers an opportunity to create a more equitable educational system.

What role should health foundations and health professions schools play in education reform, given their commitment to increasing the pool of minority students but their lack of expertise in public education? The Foundation's board of trustees raised this question when considering the Health Professions Partnership Initiative. While it expressed concern about investing in middle and high school students, it also recognized that efforts targeted at college students often came too late. The appropriate role for health foundations such as The Robert Wood Johnson Foundation appears to be in supporting the educational pipeline strategy by forming partnerships with medical schools, colleges, high schools, and secondary public schools.

At the high school level, a recent evaluation of the Health Professions Partnership Initiative stressed the importance of partnerships contributing to the general health and well-being of students and their communi-ties.[16] Those programs considered to be successful focused on both basic educational reform (such as teacher preparation in math and science ed-ucation and curriculum redesign) and career development for older, pri-marily middle and high school, students.

On a college level many students do not remain in the health pro-fessions pipeline because of poor secondary school preparation, little or no academic counseling from the pre–health education advisers, and a lack of financial support. One way to address educational barriers is to provide minority students with effective pre–health education professional advice. Students who have participated in the Minority Medical Educa-tion Program say that pre–health education advising is uneven across col-lege campuses and that advisers often discourage minority students from pursuing careers in medicine. Recognizing this as an area of importance, the Minority Medical Education Program sponsored a series of workshops in 2002 to provide pre–health education advisers with updated knowl-edge, skills, and incentives for working with minority students.

In addition to academic obstacles, financial barriers can be significant. Students in the Minority Medical Education Program often graduate from college with more than $50,000 of debt. The idea of adding more debt is often a barrier to pursuing a career in medicine. Recognizing the growing financial burdens on students, a financial seminar has been added to the curriculum.[17] This seminar is designed to provide an overview of how to manage money and how to finance a medical education. It has been so well received that a plan for expanding it to other minority college students in-terested in the health professions is being explored.

Finally, there is a need for better information and coordination. A simple search of the Internet revealed hundreds of programs aimed at in-creasing the numbers of minority students in medicine and other health professions. Some of these programs are summarized on a regional basis, yet there is no central repository where students can find out what is avail-able; nor is there a guide for how to plan when to participate in what pro-gram. Also, there is little or no coordination between programs. For example, students in the Foundation's Health Professions Partnership Ini-tiative and the Minority Medical Education Program would have benefited from better synergy between these two programs and from help in learning about other premedical and research programs.

2. *Many of the programs designed to help underrepresented minorities pursue a career in the health professions have been affected by the anti–affirmative action backlash.*

Beginning in the mid-1990s, several courts ruled that race cannot be used as a factor in admissions, and propositions were passed in California and Washington banning the use of racial preferences in admissions, hiring, and contracting.[18] These have resulted in a decrease in the number of minority applicants to medical and other health professions schools in these states.[19] Although these cases have had their biggest impact on public educational institutions, private institutions also face the same issues.

A decrease in applications to become sites for the expansion of the Minority Medical Education Program in 1999 may have been linked to medical schools' concerns that their participation might be challenged. In 1998, to allow the sites to be more inclusive, the program decided to go beyond the AAMC definition of "underrepresented minorities" (see box), which it had traditionally followed. The program now accepts all Hispanics (not just mainland Puerto Ricans and Mexican Americans) and gives each site the option of admitting a select number of students who are underrepresented in their region (Cambodians or rural whites, for example). Organizations are beginning to wrestle further with the question of what constitutes an underrepresented minority, and the AAMC is exploring a revision of its historic definition of underrepresented minorities. The issues of race and income, as well as systematic discrimination and exclusion, will be central to this discussion.

3. *Leadership is crucial to success.*

Having both minority and majority leaders strongly support the goal of increasing the numbers of minorities in the health professions has been a critical factor in achieving results. Over the decades, a large number of people the Foundation has supported have emerged as public spokespersons, as members of the Foundation's National Advisory Committees, and as leaders of academic health centers, federal government agencies, and foundations. Collectively, they have helped keep the issue of a diverse

—✲—

## *Definition of "Underrepresented Minorities"*

Over the past three decades, the definition of "underrepresented minorities" has become increasingly controversial as the population of the United States has become more diverse. The most consistently used definition of underrepresented minorities was developed by the AAMC in 1970. The AAMC defined underrepresented minorities as blacks, Mexican Americans, Native Americans (that is American Indians, Alaska Natives, and Native Hawaiians), and mainland Puerto Ricans. In 1971 the definition of minorities was modified to exclude Puerto Ricans living on the island of Puerto Rico, and in 1981 the definition was broadened to include permanent residents, as well as American citizens, who fall into these four broad categories.

The federal government has used an expanded version of this definition. With respect to the health professions, it defines underrepresented minorities as those racial and ethnic populations that are underrepresented in the health professions relative to the number of individuals who are included in the population involved. This definition includes black or African American, Hispanic or Latino, American Indian or Alaskan Native, and Native Hawaiians or other Pacific Islanders. Asians are not considered to be underrepresented minorities. In addition, many federal government programs, such as the Centers of Excellence or the Health Careers Opportunity Programs, combine the definition of underrepresented minority with the concept of disadvantage in setting the criteria for their programs. A "disadvantaged" student is defined as a student from an environment that has inhibited the individual from obtaining the knowledge, the skills, and the abilities to succeed in a health professions school or a program providing education or training in an allied health profession, *and/or* a student from a family with an annual income below a level based on low-income thresholds according to family size. Students must be U.S. citizens, noncitizen nationals, or foreign nationals with a visa permitting permanent residence in the United States.

*Sources:* http://bhpr.hrsa.gov/diversity/definitions.htm;
http://crchd.nci.nih.gov/spn/about/def.html; http://coe.stanford.edu/mingroups.html.

medical workforce on the social and health policy agenda, even in the face of mounting opposition.

Strong leaders have been instrumental in forming the partnerships that have increased the numbers of minority students pursuing careers in the health professions. Yet partnerships between health professions schools, public schools, colleges, and community agencies have been difficult to develop and sustain. The evaluation of the Health Professions Partnership Initiative identified several elements of effective partnerships. They include common goals that matter to each partner; regular communication among all partners; methods for decision making and conflict resolution; a strong leader; and the ability of each partner to commit resources. Furthermore, for programs to be effective, they must be part of the fabric of health professions schools, garnering the support of senior faculty members and administrators. Partnerships can launch a successful program, but broad leadership is required to ensure long-term stability.

The philanthropic sector also can play a leadership role by developing partnerships between health and education foundations. Such partnerships can target resources more effectively, foster working relationships between educational institutions and health professions schools, and draw attention to using evidence-based initiatives from both sectors to make change. Foundations can set an example for the larger field by coordinating their separate efforts, sharing information, and bringing more cohesion to programs. These efforts should be linked to relevant federal government programs.

4. *More rigorous evaluation of program strategies is needed.*

Measuring the results of programs to increase the numbers of minorities entering the health professions when involvement begins in high school and proceeds through college presents a number of challenges. Obviously, the outcome—entering medical school—takes place well after the initial involvement. The efforts to enhance the preparation of minority students are fragmented, programs do not follow one strategy or design, and it is difficult to attribute results to a single effort.

For the most part, knowledge about the effectiveness of minority programs comes from accumulated case studies. Taking this knowledge and using it to design more standardized evaluations presents a particularly strong challenge. For example, a significant failing of the Health Professions Partnership Initiative was its lack of attention to developing cohorts of students in each partnership program that were followed over time. The only information available derives from anecdotes and some small-scale studies that describe the success or the limitations of certain components of each program. There is no way to ascertain what combination of strategies was most effective or what the effective dose was. What is known more generally is that programs need to begin early, to be intense and sustained over time, to address nonacademic barriers, and to choose partnership institutions carefully.

Within the Minority Medical Education Program, data are available to track who applied to and entered medical school, but there are no data on what happened to student participants who did not go on to medical school. There is no tracking of whether they entered other health professions or pursued professional careers outside of health. Future programs need stronger data so that they can best determine how to use limited resources to help create a diverse and strong health professions workforce.

## —\\\\\\— The Changing Environment

Minority populations are the fastest-growing segment of the American population. By 2010, Hispanics, African Americans, Native Americans, and Asian Pacific Americans will make up 32 percent of the population, and 48 percent of the population by 2050. Health professionals need to have the cultural competence to address the health needs of diverse populations and to improve the quality of care for minority populations. The lack of providers in disadvantaged minority communities continues to be a critical impediment to health care access.

The disparity in the care received by minorities and majorities remains a significant problem, with new efforts being directed to closing the racial and ethnic gaps. In *Unequal Treatment,* a 2002 Institute of Medicine report, an argument was made for reducing disparities by increasing the number of minorities in the health care workforce and by improving the competence of the health care workforce in working with racial and ethnic populations.[20] This twofold strategy was adopted in a recent Foundation workforce program, Pipeline, Professional and Practice: Community-Based Dental Education, which is designed to address the problem of disparities in access to dental care. Under this program, which builds on a study funded by the Josiah Macy, Jr. Foundation, eleven dental schools will undertake a three-pronged strategy: finding approaches to attract low-income and minority students to attend dental schools; redesigning the dental schools' curricula to make them more relevant to community-based practice; and creating accessible dental services sites in the communities. The Kellogg Foundation is providing scholarship support for minority students attending the eleven dental schools. Based on the Foundation's model, the California Endowment is funding programs in four additional California dental schools and also will be providing scholarship support.

Of course, the national debate over affirmative action affects educational programs that seek to promote a more diverse health care workforce. The U.S. Supreme Court handed down two decisions in June 2003 regarding the University of Michigan's undergraduate and law school admissions policies. The Court held that diversity in the student body is a compelling interest that can justify the use of race as a plus factor in admissions decisions. It found in favor of Michigan Law School's practice of giving individualized consideration to all applicants in order to achieve a "critical mass" of underrepresented minorities. At the same time, it struck down the undergraduate admissions policy that awarded extra points to minority applicants.

The message from these decisions is that in the admissions process, only individualized consideration that gives substantial weight to diversity factors other than race will be constitutional. This will present challenges to universities seeking diverse student bodies since such tailored approaches will be difficult for the many undergraduate programs that receive thousands of applications every year. Affirmative action admissions systems will be subject to case-by-case challenges. These have often been successful in the past, although with the guidance given by the Supreme Court, universities may be able to craft programs that will withstand the challenges.

Despite court challenges and ballot initiatives, momentum has been building to create a diverse health workforce. In August 1996, the AAMC created a coalition of Health Professionals for Diversity. Made up of more than thirty of the nation's leading medical, health, and education associations, the coalition serves as an advocate for the continued use of race, ethnicity, and gender as factors in the admissions process. In 1998, a Pew Health Professions Commission released a report calling for a major increase in racial, ethnic, and socioeconomic diversity in the health care workforce.[21] The report warned that without such diversity health professionals in the twenty-first century would be poorly equipped to care for an increasingly diverse population.

Many other organizations have made the case for diversity in the health care workforce. Jordan Cohen, president of the AAMC, and his colleagues articulated the case cogently. Writing in *Health Affairs* in 2002, they argued that adequate representation among students and faculty of the diversity in American society was indispensable for quality medical education; that increasing the diversity of the physician workforce would improve access to health care for underserved populations; that increasing the diversity of the research workforce could accelerate advances in medical and public health research; and that diversity among managers of health care organizations made good business sense.[22]

## —ɯ— Conclusion

The promise of the 1960s to solve our nation's racial and ethnic inequalities has not been realized. Despite the large amount of resources invested, underrepresented minorities constitute only 10.6 percent of physicians, 5 percent of dentists, and 12.3 percent of nurses. Yet the 2000 census data reveal that over 25 percent of the U.S. population is African American, Hispanic, or Native American/Alaskan Native, and these percentages are growing rapidly. Thus, persistent underrepresentation of minorities in the health professions remains a major challenge.

Meeting the challenge—that is, developing a health professions workforce that looks like the general population—goes well beyond issues of access to, or cultural competence in, health care. It touches on society's obligation to eliminate educational inequities that harm the health, well-being, and potential of large numbers of our citizens. Now more than ever, programs that address the educational barriers faced by minorities must be protected and strengthened.

## Notes

1. For this chapter, *minority* is used to mean underrepresented minorities except where otherwise noted.

2. *Changing the Face of Medicine: Celebrating Fifty Years (1946–1996).* National Medical Fellowships, Inc., 1997.

3. *Report of the Association of American Medical Colleges Task Force on Minority Student Opportunities in Medicine.* June 1978.

4. In general, a foundation is required to make grants amounting to 5 percent of its assets each year to qualify for tax-exempt status.

5. Isaacs, S. L., Sandy, L. G., and Schroeder, S. A. "Improving the Health Care Workforce: Perspectives from Twenty-Four Years' Experience." In *To Improve Health and Health Care 1997: The Robert Wood Johnson Foundation Anthology.* San Francisco: Jossey-Bass, 1997.

6. Baratz, J., and Keyser-Smith, J. *Report to the Robert Wood Johnson Foundation: Expanding Medical Education Opportunities for Minority Students.* Educational Policy Research Institute, Educational Testing Service, Mar. 1982.

7. Keyser-Smith, J. *Black Participation in Engineering Education.* Washington, D.C.: Educational Policy Research Institute, Oct. 1981.

8. Bridges, K., and Smith, L. *Evaluation Report to The Robert Wood Johnson Foundation on the Minority Medical Faculty Development Program.* (Unpublished). 1995.

9. *National Program Report: Minority Medical Faculty Development Program.* The Robert Wood Johnson Foundation, July 2001. (www.rwjf.org/reports/npreports/mfde.htm).

10. Cantor, J. C., Bergeisen, L., and Baker, L. "Effect of Intensive Educational Program for Minority College Students and Recent Graduates on the Probability of Acceptance to Medical School." *JAMA,* 1998, *280,* 772–776.

11. Ready, T., and Nickens, H. W. "Programs That Make a Difference." In B. H. Kehrer and H. C. Burroughs (eds.), *More Minorities in Health.* Menlo Park, Calif.: The Henry Kaiser Family Foundation, 1994.

12. Lewin, M. *The Foundation's Minority Medical Training Programs.* Special Report, The Robert Wood Johnson Foundation, 1987.

13. Petersdorf, R. G. "Not a Choice, an Obligation." *Academic Medicine,* 1992, *67,* 73–79.

14. Association of American Medical Colleges. "Special Theme Issue: Educational Programs to Strengthen the Medical School Pipeline." *Academic Medicine,* 1999, *74,* 305–460.

15. Darling-Hammond, L. "Inequality in Teaching and Schooling: How Opportunity Is Rationed to Students of Color in America." In B. D. Smedley, A. Y. Stith, L. Colburn, and C. H. Evans (eds.), *The Right Thing to Do, the Smart Thing to Do.* Washington, D.C.: National Academy Press, 2001, pp. 208–233; Gandara, P. "Lost Opportunities: The Difficult Journey to Higher Education." In B. D. Smedley, A. Y. Stith, L. Colburn, and C. H. Evans (eds.), *The Right Thing to Do, the Smart Thing to Do.* Washington, D.C.: National Academy Press, 2001, pp. 234–259.

16. Carline, J. D., and Patterson, D. G. *Assessment of the Health Professions Partnership Initiative: A Report to the Robert Wood Johnson Foundation.* Aug. 2002.

17. Terrell, C., Bletzinger, R., and Ficklen, E. "A Financial Planning Workshop for Minority Students." *Transcript,* 2003, *14,* 44–47.

18. Perez, T. E. "Current Legal Status of Affirmative Action Programs in Higher Education." In B. D. Smedley, A. Y. Stith, L. Colburn, and C. H. Evans (eds.), *The Right Thing to Do, the Smart Thing to Do.* Washington, D.C.: National Academy Press, 2001, pp. 91–116.

19. Grumbach, K., Coffman, J., Rosenoff, E., and Munoz, C. "Trends in Underrepresented Minority Participation in Health Professions Schools." In B. D. Smedley, A. Y. Stith, L. Colburn, and C. H. Evans (eds.), *The Right Thing to Do, the Smart Thing to Do.* Washington, D.C.: National Academy Press, 2001, pp. 185–207.

20. Smedley, B., Stith, A., and Nelson, A. *Unequal Treatment: Confronting Racial and Ethnic Disparities in Health Care.* Washington, D.C.: National Academy Press, 2002.

21. *Recreating Health Professional Practice for a New Century.* Pew Health Professions Commission, Dec. 1998.

22. Cohen, J., Gabriel, B., and Terrell, C. "The Case for Diversity in the Health Care Workforce." *Health Affairs,* Sept.-Oct. 2002, pp. 90–102.

# The National Health Policy Forum

*Richard S. Frank*

## Editors' Introduction

Given the importance of the federal government to The Robert Wood Johnson Foundation's mission of improving the health and health care of all Americans, it is natural for the Foundation to try to make sure that those who shape health policy do so on the basis of the most current and accurate information. Currently, the Foundation has 219 active grants, totaling $257 million, designed to improve policy-relevant information and to enrich the dialogue that is a key part of the policymaking process. These include support for the journal *Health Affairs,* for studies coordinated by the Institute of Medicine, for a health policy fellowship program, and for a new program that synthesizes research findings into short policy-relevant reports.

In this chapter Richard S. Frank, the former editor of *National Journal* and now an adjunct professor of journalism at Boston University's Washington Journalism Center, discusses the National Health Policy Forum, which the Foundation has supported since 1973. The Forum offers a seminar series on emerging health policy issues for elected officials, members of the executive branch, administrative agency officials, and their staffs.

Striving to be politically neutral, the Forum provides high-quality nonpartisan information and analysis that allow different viewpoints to be heard. (Its approach is similar to that of The Robert Wood Johnson Foundation, which is committed to improving health care and health status, but typically avoids taking positions on partisan issues and specific health policy solutions.) Frank assesses whether being a neutral convener is sufficient in an era of great partisanship.

The Foundation has funded similar health policy forums in a number of states. These state-based forums are advancing a growing field devoted to translating research into practice and synthesizing complicated and sometimes contradictory research findings into formats useful to policymakers.

—ɱ—      In many ways, the room, in a Washington hotel a few blocks from the Capitol, resembles a large university lecture hall, filled with students ready to absorb some scholarly information and insight. But many of the 150 people gathered here are not in fact students but are senior aides and advisers to some of the most influential and powerful health policymakers in the federal government. Roughly half of them work on Capitol Hill or in the executive branch, in approximately equal numbers.

They are attending a National Health Policy Forum session on Medicare's role in paying for the care of the chronically ill. That may not be as politically potent a subject as, for example, how the government should help older Americans pay for the soaring costs of prescription medicine. But it is an issue that policymakers—and particularly their principal aides and advisers—will almost certainly have to understand and deal with when they finally come to grips with the critically important issue of how to keep Medicare financially healthy as the population ages.

Many of the attendees obviously know one another, and as they munch on the buffet lunch offered before the formal session, they exchange personal and professional notes. Others peer at name tags and introduce themselves. A few pull others aside to recommend a new research report or project.

Those present at the early-spring session hear two experts from outside the government and three federal health specialists devote two hours during the middle of a busy day to discussing the problems associated with the increasing percentage of Medicare beneficiaries who have chronic medical conditions. It is the kind of topic and the kind of setting that has identified the National Health Policy Forum since its inception three decades ago. The Forum today remains what it set out to be in 1971: a resource for informal and private exchange of information and ideas about health policy among congressional and executive agency staff members. That's particularly important, its leaders say, at a time when official Washington's interest in health policy issues has burgeoned while the expertise of the congressional and executive branch staffs has diminished, in large measure because of increasingly high turnover rates on Capitol Hill.

Stuart Altman, now a professor of national health policy at Brandeis University, was there at the beginning. As a deputy assistant secretary at the old Department of Health, Education and Welfare, he was one of fewer than two dozen health policy specialists working on Capitol Hill and in the executive branch who gathered for dinner one evening in 1971 to launch a series of informal seminars on important issues in their subject area. These seminars soon developed into the National Health Policy Forum. Altman says that the Forum, or something very much like it, continues to be necessary as a way of dealing with the explosive growth of the health policy debate in Washington. In fact, he says, the increasingly partisan tone of the debate may mean that "a neutral voice is needed more than ever."

The Forum has tried to position itself as a neutral voice from the day it began. Its guiding principle—never to advocate a particular policy and never to take a stand on specific legislation—is intact. But the Forum today confronts some notable paradoxes. The rapid expansion of federal health policy over the years, which should surely be expected to enhance the role of a program dedicated to informing health policymakers, has kept senior congressional health policy aides so busy that they have less time than ever to attend Forum seminars or to read Forum materials. Similarly, in an era of often bitter divisiveness, both ideological and partisan, on most health policy issues, the Forum's neutrality may not meet the needs of those who are seeking solutions rather than options.

So should the Forum seek to carve out a new role for itself by becoming more of a player—though never a partisan one—by actively developing and perhaps even brokering solutions? Those who lead and advise the Forum respond that adopting such a role would be a serious mistake.

The Forum's Web site proudly proclaims that since it began, it has conducted more than eight hundred workshops, technical briefings, and site visits. It has also produced more than eight hundred background papers and what it calls "Issue Briefs," the not-so-brief summaries of the issues that are the Forum's trademark. Its annual budget had grown to $3.1 million in 2002, of which 90 percent came from foundations, with The Robert Wood Johnson Foundation (27 percent), the David and Lucile Packard Foundation (23 percent), and the W. K. Kellogg Foundation (19 percent) accounting for the largest shares of support. The Robert Wood Johnson Foundation, in fact, has been sufficiently pleased by the Forum's accomplishments that it has awarded grants to half a dozen state programs that are similar in approaches and goals to those of the Forum (see box).

After three decades, the Forum is clearly a survivor. But can it continue to be effective, given its determination to stand apart from what it has described as "the highly charged politics of Capitol Hill"?[1] In a harshly divided national capital, is impartiality enough? The Forum's answer: for the good of the public policy system, it had better be.

## —∿— Getting Started

Informed neutrality was the Forum's goal from its inception. In 1971, Medicare and Medicaid were only six years old, but Congress was already beginning to fine-tune these two huge government programs. Health care, though not the ascendant political issue it has since become, was already looming as a major congressional subject. To Altman and his colleagues in the executive and legislative branches, it was imperative that they—and through them, their principals in the Nixon administration and in Congress—have the information they needed to make sound policy judgments.

With a Republican in the White House and Democrats in control of Congress, the health policy aides found themselves working in a climate of political distrust. And with the executive agencies as the primary source of information on health care, many congressional Democrats were starting to express doubts about the objectivity of that information. One solution that seemed to appeal to some of these aides was already being tried out in the field of education policy: Why not bring congressional and executive health policy staffs together to exchange information and views and—perhaps as important—to try to break down the walls, real or imaginary, that appeared to divide them?

A program called the Educational Staff Seminar had been functioning for several years, holding meetings in Washington and conducting occasional out-of-town site visits. It seemed a likely model for the health policy specialists to adopt and adapt. (In fact, the organization that ultimately became the National Health Policy Forum was known in its early years as the Health Staff Seminar.) After all, Washington was spending much more on health than on education, Judith Miller Jones, the Forum's director, recalled in a recent interview. Jones, at the time a legislative liaison for the Department of Health, Education and Welfare (now the Department of Health and Human Services), was one of the Educational Staff Seminar participants. She was asked to help Altman and the other health policy specialists write a planning grant application to the Carnegie Corporation of New York to get the program started. It was officially launched under the auspices of The George Washington University, which has been its sponsor ever since.

The start-up grant from Carnegie allowed the new group to hire a small staff, and Jones became its first—and only—director. Her experience at the time was limited to a year at the Department of Health, Education and Welfare and two years as an aide to Senator Winston Prouty, a Vermont Republican, for whom she specialized in education and, as she recalled, "a little bit" of health policy. In 1973, The Robert Wood Johnson Foundation provided a small sum for a study to determine whether it should help the new group financially. It decided to do so "and took us under its wing," Jones said. Initially, the Foundation awarded the Forum a three-year grant of $498,000. It subsequently became the Forum's major supporter and has so far provided it with slightly more than $10 million in grants.

From the beginning the Forum's mission has been to offer "a unique, off-the-record setting for interaction and exchange of ideas, removed from the highly charged politics of Capitol Hill." The group's organizers, Jones recalled, made an early decision not to seek or accept federal money for the program, as had the Educational Staff Seminar, and therefore not to become beholden financially to the executive branch.

But while the Forum has not sought federal financial help, the inclusion of executive branch aides has always been an important part of the Forum's philosophy. In fact, about 40 percent of the members of the Forum's policy-setting Steering Committee are from executive branch agencies. An equal number are legislative aides, with staff members of congressional support agencies filling the rest of the committee's slots.

## —⟋⟍— A Different Audience

The heart of the Forum's program has always been its seminars—almost always off the record—on important but sometimes arcane issues of health care policy. The Forum's intention from the start was to bring senior congressional and executive staffs together to discuss these issues while carefully sidestepping any temptation to offer political advice. Outside policy experts and real-world practitioners are regularly invited to present their views to the legislative and administrative staffs and to join in discussing the subject.

"When this program got started, we were all terribly naïve," Jones said. Medicare and Medicaid were both still in their infancy, she pointed out, and policymakers "didn't really understand the links between money and health care," such as how doctors and hospitals are paid, the role of insurers, and how the two vast new federal programs were driving costs. "We didn't yet grasp just how health care delivery systems were affected by these huge dollar flows."

The Forum has undoubtedly lost its naïveté since 1971. It has also lost part of its audience during the past three decades—a loss that poses questions about the program's continued vitality.

Historically, the staff members of the congressional committees and subcommittees responsible for health policy made up the Forum's core audience.[2] But as the health policy workload and complexity have increased, these staff members have found it increasingly difficult to keep on top of all the issues. At the same time, for many of the aides on the personal staffs of committee members, health policy is only one of several subjects in their work portfolio, and these aides necessarily lack the specialized expertise of committee staff members. Moreover, staff turnover is a problem; the Forum has noted that many congressional aides "use their Hill experience as a stepping stone to a remunerative lobbying or trade association position."[3]

Staff turnover, whatever the cause, has required the Forum to make some adjustments. For example, Jones said, when the Democrats took control of the Senate in 2001, the health staff of the Senate Finance

Committee asked the Forum to brief it on the Health Care Financing Administration's governance role on Medicare and Medicaid. The Forum responded with four briefings and a site visit. In the fall of 2002, Jones said, the committee staff members asked for help in running briefings on the fundamentals of the Medicare and Medicaid programs for new health policy aides, perhaps on an annual basis. They asked for the briefings on such a basic subject, Jones said, "because they recognized that high turnover was hurting their productivity."

So, for example, on January 23 and 24, 2003, the Forum held an invitation-only seminar titled "Understanding Medicare and Medicaid: Fundamentals and Issues for the New Congress," with a voluminous "electronic briefing book" on the subject—links to various documents, charts, and PowerPoint presentations. The session, which the Forum said on its Web site was "requested by congressional staff to provide an overview of the Medicare, Medicaid, and State Children's Health Insurance programs," was clearly a response to the turnover problem. But "basic training" sessions like that may risk diminishing the Forum's relevance as the source of leading-edge policy information.

The growth of staff positions in congressional support agencies— the General Accounting Office, the Congressional Budget Office, and the Library of Congress's Congressional Research Service—has helped to compensate for the decline in the size of committee staffs. Many of the support agency aides with expertise in health policy expect to stay in their positions "indefinitely," the Forum has pointed out. Meanwhile, participation by executive agency staffs has continued, and, as a consequence, "the Forum's audience has become larger and more diverse than in the days when Hill staff dominated Forum activities."[4]

Whether that diversity serves the Forum's goals has been the subject of some debate. "We now serve the congressional [support] agencies as our lead audience," Jones said during the interview. "They come to our meetings, and then, in turn, they brief the newer, less experienced congressional committee staffs. That's a big change. It's like training the trainers."

A particular concern of some observers of the Forum's work is that the most influential people on Capitol Hill may be staying away from the off-the-record policy seminars. "The Forum will maximize its influence to the extent it is attended by individuals (or its materials are read by individuals) who are likely to influence policy," concluded a 1997 assessment of the Forum conducted for The Robert Wood Johnson Foundation by New Directions for Policy, a Washington-based policy research, analysis, and strategic planning firm. Linda Fishman, the health policy director of the Republican staff of the Senate Finance Committee and a member of the Forum's Steering Committee, agreed that for senior congressional aides "it's very hard to break away" to attend the often lengthy seminars. Linda T. Bilheimer, who, as a Congressional Budget Office official, served on the Forum's Steering Committee until she moved to The Robert Wood Johnson Foundation at the end of 1999, assigns the blame to high congressional turnover. "The senior, experienced staff are stretched unbelievably thin," she said. "So for them, getting away to meetings is extremely hard." For the inexperienced staff, on the other hand, "the level of the material may be too hard for them because the Forum pitches to quite a sophisticated audience."

Bilheimer, now the Foundation's senior program officer monitoring the Forum, said that the Forum was getting requests to provide "more basic education on the Hill," not necessarily at the regular seminars but instead at separate sessions for various committee staffs. She said that doing this would preserve the high level of sophistication at the seminars while offering basic education on health care policy for the less experienced. Senior Hill aides, Bilheimer suggested, would come to special, restricted-attendance meetings if they were held in addition to the larger meetings. Whether justified or not, she said, the senior staff members believe they get more out of "meeting with a small group of their peers than being in a larger group."

The 1997 evaluation report pointed to another irony: that the Issue Briefs distributed before every seminar were such good summaries of the subject that their very excellence "may detract from attendance at the meetings." Bilheimer is skeptical. She acknowledged that while she was at the Congressional Budget Office, where she was the deputy assistant director for health, she "always appreciated the quality of the Issue Briefs, because it meant that if I couldn't go to a meeting, I had the documents at hand." "But," she added, "I did try to go to meetings if I could because the Forum has done a good job of bringing in speakers who aren't the usual suspects. And I often found that I could hear viewpoints expressed at the meetings that greatly enriched the materials that were available in the Issue Briefs."

Jones agreed that some Capitol Hill health policy specialists may be too busy to attend the seminars. She noted that some of them call the Forum office to find out what happened at a meeting they had missed. On the other hand, she said, others want to come to a meeting "to see how other people are facing the issue. They want to schmooze." Jones also pointed out that the Issue Briefs, along with the Forum's lengthier background papers, are available at the organization's Web site.

## —ᴡᴡ— Touchy Topics

Most health policy subjects worth considering are certain to be controversial. For a program that's determined to preserve its neutrality, the Forum's challenge is to avoid controversy while concentrating on deeply contentious topics. It must also strive to be timely without slavishly adhering to anyone's legislative or administrative agenda.

The narrow line the Forum must walk requires that it choose its topics carefully and then develop and present information that's useful but nonprescriptive. The Forum's Steering Committee has the dominant role in deciding what to look at; the Forum's staff is responsible for the way the topic is presented.

The Forum's staff periodically presents the Steering Committee with a list of proposed activities—seminars and other meetings in Washington and site visits to other locales—for the next twelve months. The committee, which has approximately forty members who work for members of Congress, congressional committees and support organizations, and executive agencies, then accepts, rejects, or modifies items on the list. So, for example, a list prepared in September 2002 included thirty-three proposed activities. This list, which gives a sense of the range of issues the Forum typically has on its calendar, included these activities:

- A meeting and Issue Brief on "Medicare's Prospective Payment Systems: In Sync or in Disarray?"

- An Issue Brief on prescription drug use in nursing homes
- A site visit to Phoenix to examine "The Medicare and Medicaid Intersection: Caring for Arizona's Seniors"
- A primer on long-term care insurance
- A meeting and Issue Brief updating a similar session and brief in 2001 on "The State Budget Crisis: How Have Health Programs Fared?"
- A "seniors only" meeting to discuss "Waiting for the Next Vision: Purchasing Health Care in Uncertain Times"
- A meeting and Issue Brief on "Emergency Medical Response for a Mass Casualty Event"

Sometimes, according to Jones, "the committee will say, 'This is a terribly important issue, but put it later because other things have come up that we have to get to sooner.' Other things, they tell us, 'Move it up on the agenda.'"

At one time, Jones said, the Forum had an external advisory board to guide it in its selection of topics. "But the Steering Committee members said they didn't want any outsiders 'telling us what we need to look at. We know what we need to know, and we're not going to have them veto what we say.'"

Steering Committee member Fishman said that Jones "listens to health staff" in choosing topics. "We identify what are the hot topics. We'll say, 'Gee, that needs to be pushed up, we need to know that sooner, that one is less important, wait on that one.' We identify what's important, the hot topics, the things we need information on right away" because legislation on the subject is before Congress.

Bilheimer views the process as "sort of a two-way street. The Forum staff generates ideas for topics," and the Steering Committee responds. When she was a Steering Committee member, she recalled recently, "we would go to meetings, and a very lengthy list of potential topics would be produced" by the Forum staff. "And the committee would say, 'We think this is the greatest thing since sliced bread,' or 'We don't quite understand where you're going with this one,' and would cull down to the ones we thought were really important. We would also raise ideas for topics that we thought were important." Moreover, she said, if the key people on a committee staff said that they saw the need to study a particular topic, "the Forum staff would jump" and add that topic to the agenda.

## —w— Rejecting Outside Influence

In deciding which issues to put on its calendar, the Forum staff is aware of the interests and goals of its primary financing sources, The Robert Wood Johnson Foundation, the David and Lucile Packard Foundation, and the W. K. Kellogg Foundation. But Jones, Bilheimer, and program officers for the other foundations agree that they don't dictate the subject of specific Forum topics.

Packard's primary interest in the health policy arena involves issues of children's health. It encourages the Forum to come up with topics in that area, said Eugene Lewit, the foundation's senior program manager for the Forum. But he added that Packard avoids recommending specific subjects to the Forum.

Barbara Sabol, program director for the Forum at Kellogg, explained in an interview that the Forum each year submits a proposal that states what it intends to focus on that year. Kellogg comments on the list, she said, and also keeps the Forum informed of what the foundation is up to. One of Kellogg's objectives is "to get feedback on national policies," Sabol said. And though health care is not Kellogg's major area of interest, "there are a lot of cross-cutting issues involved, such as education, in which child health care plays an important part. So what the Forum does relates to many of our issues."

From the very beginning, Jones said, Robert Wood Johnson Foundation officials insisted that the Forum avoid any appearance that they were driving its agenda. The Foundation staff told her, she recalled, "We're not going to control what you do, because it's tremendously important that people see this as a safe haven, where they can learn from each other." She added that the Foundation's grant to the Forum "is written in such a way that they know we're going to cover the waterfront. We also know what their priority areas are."

For the Foundation, the Forum meets a very particular need, Bilheimer said, and while the Foundation has broader health policy interests than the Forum has, it deals with those interests in other ways. From time to time, she explained, the Foundation will tell the Forum staff that "we think it would be helpful" for the Forum to have a meeting on a specific topic. And sometimes Bilheimer will tell the Forum staff that other Foundation grantees have been working in a subject area "that it might be really interesting to have a Forum session on." If the Forum staff chooses not to add the topic to its agenda, that's fine with the Foundation, she said, adding that even if the staff likes the subject, the Steering Committee has to agree.

The Forum has, in fact, responded negatively on one subject dear to the Foundation: behavioral issues such as alcohol and drug abuse and smoking. Over the years, the Foundation has encouraged the Forum to conduct meetings and prepare Issue Briefs on the topic, and from time to time the Forum has done that, according to Jones. But the Forum, she added, has also told the Foundation that "such issues are not high-priority to most of the audience and tend to attract the already convinced. And there are limits to what people think government can and should do, especially at the federal level, while foundations have a much broader array of options to support."

Nevertheless, the Forum depends on the money it gets from foundations, and if a major contributor is interested in a particular broad subject, the Forum is going to be especially cautious about ignoring it. The Forum's lone complaint about its relationship with The Robert Wood Johnson Foundation, Jones said, "is one we have never solved. They expect us to read their minds and know everything that they're doing. And if we don't mention it, we get blamed." This has been a problem for thirty years, she said. "Does the Foundation want to control things? No. Do they want to maximize impact by having everybody on the same wavelength? Sure. As much as possible."

Foundations other than Robert Wood Johnson, Packard, and Kellogg—the Forum also receives grants from the California HealthCare Foundation, the Flinn Foundation, the John A. Hartford Foundation, and the John D. and Catherine T. MacArthur Foundation—make fewer demands on the Forum's agenda.

The Forum also receives money from corporations with strong business interests in health policy. It tries to avoid any hint of improper influence, Jones said, by limiting total corporate contributions to about 1 percent of the Forum's budget, by declining grants for specific purposes, and by mingling the corporate gifts with its other revenue. The Forum has received corporate support from pharmaceutical companies such as GlaxoSmithKline, Johnson & Johnson, Merck, and Pfizer; health insurers such as Blue Cross Blue Shield, Kaiser Permanente, and UnitedHealth Group; and other health-related companies.

Accepting corporate grants "came about by accident," Jones said, when the Forum was studying health insurance and she went to the Prudential Insurance Company of America for some information. Prudential offered her what she described as "a token amount of money." She went to her Steering Committee, which decided, in her words, that if insurance companies were part of the problem, "they ought to be part of the solution."

Only once, Jones said, has a corporation "tried to manipulate us." That was a drug company, which she declined to identify and which no longer exists, whose money was returned. She added that a foundation tried the same thing and was dealt with in the same way.

## —ᨮ— Balancing Act

After getting its marching orders from the Steering Committee, the Forum staff of about twenty organizes the meetings and site visits and puts together, sometimes with the help of outside writers, the multipage Issue Briefs, the even longer background papers, and the reports on Forum site visits. Whether the staff writes the papers depends on its expertise on the subject, Jones said. If necessary, she will employ freelance writers, including two former staff members who write regularly for the Forum. "We also have a few stringers we use," she said. "And we pay them well. But you can't continue a program with just stringers." Moreover, she said, some former contributors turned in work that the Forum wouldn't publish.

"It's a problem we'll never be able to fix," Jones said. One reason for the difficulty, she pointed out, is that some of the outside writers "aren't used to writing in a nonpartisan, objective way" and that some of them "are advocates at heart."

How successful are the Forum's writers—in-house or outside—in avoiding the extremes of cold-blooded neutrality and warm-blooded advocacy? A review of some recent Issue Briefs suggests that they have struck the appropriate balance between identifying and analyzing a problem and recommending a course of action. Two recent Issue Briefs might also serve as examples of how to handle political hot potatoes without any risk of burning hands or mouth.

In June 2002, the Forum published an Issue Brief titled *Average Wholesale Price for Prescription Drugs: Is There a More Appropriate Pricing Mechanism?* The brief carefully sidesteps endorsing any particular solution to the important and politically sensitive problem of prescription drug pricing while making it clear that the average wholesale price mechanism has major defects. Its concluding paragraph is worth quoting in full as an example of the Forum's approach:

> The AWP [average wholesale price], a pricing mechanism that by most accounts is seriously flawed and not widely understood, plays a pivotal role in the overall prescription drug pricing and reimbursement systems. It has become a critical benchmark for key stakeholders, despite its inability to accurately reflect the "true cost" of drugs. Yet, as we have seen, the true cost of a given drug depends on the various discounts, rebates, and reimbursement formulas available to a particular purchaser—both public and private. Other alternatives to the AWP may suffer from similar flaws, namely, being subject to manipulation and not closely aligned with real market transaction prices. The creation of an appropriate payment mechanism for prescription drugs, therefore, will need to involve a careful balance between protecting the proprietary nature of drug pricing information and ensuring the accuracy of, and accountability for, the information on which such a payment mechanism is based.[5]

Three months later another Issue Brief, titled *Medigap: Prevalence, Premiums, and Opportunities for Reform,* comes even closer to the line between descriptive and prescriptive without crossing it. It ends this way:

Budget constraints mean that the tension between providing catastrophic coverage to the sickest beneficiaries and first-dollar coverage for those who are risk-averse will likely worsen with time. In light of changes to retiree health insurance plans and M + C [Medicare + Choice] plans, the time seems ripe to reconsider whether the Medigap market is fulfilling policymakers' goals and expectations.[6]

As for its goal of timeliness, the Forum was reacting to Congress's scramble to meet a recently revealed need when it published an Issue Brief in June 2002 with the title *Will the Nation Be Ready for the Next Bioterrorism Attack? Mending Gaps in the Public Health Infrastructure.* The Issue Brief's baleful conclusion: "Fortifying the public health infrastructure will clearly be a long-term endeavor. . . . The potential for a real reform of public health preparedness capabilities will depend on the sustained involvement and commitment of policymakers at all levels of government. Close scrutiny must be paid to determine what is working, what is not, and what additional measures need to be pursued."[7]

In asking The Robert Wood Johnson Foundation in 1999 to renew its grant, the Forum had this to say about its policy mission: "While the Forum never takes positions on political proposals under debate, we believe that our activities often make the debates more informed and knowledge-based than they otherwise would be."[8]

Not everyone agrees with that position, however. In the 1997 evaluation of the Forum, several congressional aides suggested to the evaluators that the seminars could be more useful if they discussed legislative solutions more directly. While that suggestion falls short of a demand to propose solutions, it is clearly a call for the program to present an array of possible solutions even if it doesn't single one out for recommendation.

The Steering Committee's Fishman, for one, takes issue with the suggestion. The Forum, she said, "tries to be straight-shooting presenters of information without having a point of view." It needs to pay attention to the hot legislative topics, she added, "but not in a partisan way."

Jones has equally strong views on the subject. "Some people wanted us to recommend solutions," she said. "But the Steering Committee said no, because the moment you do that you alienate one side or the other." Offering solutions, she added, is "what lobbyists are paid to do." After the

Republicans captured control of the House in the 1994 elections, "we were the only program that was still seen as neutral," Jones said. "Every other program was seen as tainted by one side or the other." Admittedly, Jones said, some senior people call the Forum from time to time to ask what the staff thinks about a particular legislative proposal. "We'll respond," she said. "But we have to be very careful that we don't look like lobbyists."

Politics and political wrangling are inescapable, of course, in discussing almost any kind of health care legislation. The Forum has tried to cope with the problem in a variety of ways.

In the fall of 1998, the Forum wrote in its annual progress report to The Robert Wood Johnson Foundation that during the previous twelve months "it became clear that the divisiveness in Washington and changes in the policy apparatus and legislative process demand new ways of doing business."[9] That was not the last time it would sound the alarm about Washington's growing political rancor.

In its report to the Foundation in 2000, the Forum observed that "the increased practice of 'coalition politics' by powerful Washington lobbyists, whereby interest groups continually realign to apply political pressure on members of Congress, often means that policy concerns are driven underground by political machinations." The report goes on to discuss the Forum's role in the policy debate: "Despite the poisonous atmosphere that such tactics often create, it is ironic that their prevalence in the current era actually underscores the need for a nonpartisan, objective forum to examine the merits of legislative proposals. The National Health Policy Forum, of course, has played this role for almost three decades."[10]

The same report also offers a pair of pointed examples of the Forum's role and the influence of politics on the way the Forum does its work. In both cases, the Forum acted as a facilitator—trying to help others to achieve their goals.

One of them involved the politically sensitive question of whether Medicare should move away from administered pricing toward more competitive pricing in buying medical services, particularly those provided by managed care plans. In the fall of 1999, with Congress deadlocked over whether to conduct demonstration projects on the subject, key congressional and executive branch aides asked the Forum to organize a small, off-the-record session "to promote dialogue among the key players" on the issue, according to the Forum's annual report. The meeting, hosted by senior Republicans on the staff of the Senate Finance Committee, was attended by other senior congressional aides and by high-ranking administration officials. The result, the Forum report says, was that key congressional staff, previously reluctant to become involved in the subject, changed their minds and became engaged. Ultimately, however, Congress decided against taking any action on the issue.[11]

The Forum, in the same report, offered another illustration of its role as facilitator. As part of its effort to examine the effects on hospital-based health systems of the 1997 Balanced Budget Act and legislation that followed it, the Forum conducted site visits in March and April 2000 to Richmond, Virginia, Detroit, and Seattle, followed by a two-day conference in Annapolis, Maryland, at the end of April. Holding so many out-of-Washington sessions in such a short time was a serious drain on the Forum's time and limited budget. So why did it undertake this resource-straining project? According to the Forum's progress report, congressional health aides wanted to be armed with sufficient information to beat back lobbyists' attempts to carve out federal health funds for their clients and pressed the Forum to accelerate its efforts to come up with that information. As the Forum observed in its report, "scheduling meetings has become an increasingly political matter."[12]

## —⚹— A Role for the Forum

Capitol Hill certainly has no shortage of information on health policy issues. Lobbyists, think tanks, and congressional research offices provide an almost endless flood of information on the issues, large and small, that Congress has to contend with. But information provided by a group without a stake in the outcome is uncommon, the Forum's defenders say, and sometimes priceless. Even more important, they add, is its closely related mission of bringing congressional and executive branch health policy staffs together, out of the political spotlight, to exchange views and get to know their policy counterparts. In an era of partisan and ideological division, that's the role the Forum is determined to play: to be a facilitator, not a broker of agreements.

"The way things are today, there's no role" for the Forum in trying to offer specific solutions or even a range of possible solutions, said Charles (Chip) Kahn III, the president of the Federation of American Hospitals and former staff director of the House Ways and Means Health Subcommittee. "I don't think that would be sustainable," given "the sharp partisan divide" in Congress today. The Forum's proper role, he said in an interview, should combine providing information and bringing opposing sides together.

The Kellogg Foundation's Barbara Sabol agrees: "I think it's imperative that there be places where one can have discussions about the issues that are not adversarial. They don't necessarily have to agree with each other, but the facts can be examined in a nonpartisan way."

That is no easy assignment. But Forum officials say they are convinced that it is at least as pertinent today as it was when the organization was born three decades ago. Jones put it succinctly in a recent interview. Some people, she said, want to know only their side of an issue, while others want to understand the issue. "They're the ones who ask, 'How do I sort it out?' We appeal to the latter."

---

—∽∾—

### A Model for the States

In 1992, the League of Women Voters of New Jersey approached The Robert Wood Johnson Foundation with an idea and a request for funds to carry it out. The League had only recently sponsored a conference in Princeton to examine health care issues and had come away from it convinced that some sort of permanent structure was needed to keep the state legislature informed of policy developments in the health field.

The Foundation said it would help and urged the League to take as its model the well-established National Health Policy Forum, which the Foundation had by then been underwriting for almost two decades. The League agreed and used the money to create the Capitol Forums on Health and Medical Care. The objective: to provide New Jersey legislators and other decision makers with non-partisan analysis and research. The League decided to withdraw from sponsorship, but the New Jersey forums have continued, with financial help from the Foundation, under the auspices of the Forums Institute for Public Policy.

Then, in 1996, the Foundation paid for a study of the feasibility of replicating the New Jersey program in other states. The study's recommendation: the Foundation should invite six states to submit proposals to develop programs by the fall of 1998 that would be patterned after the National Health Policy Forum. To that end, the Forums Institute established the State Forums Partnership Program, which offers technical assistance and onetime matching grants of up to $125,000 over three years for new state forums. The New Jersey program, by contrast, operates under renewable grants.

In the spring of 2003, the state partners were the Massachusetts Health Policy Forum at Brandeis University; the Center for Health Services Research at the University of Tennessee Health Science Center in Memphis; the Kansas Health Institute in Topeka; the Wisconsin Public Health and Health Policy Institute at the University of Wisconsin–Madison Medical School; the Texas Institute for Health Policy Research; and the Health Policy Analysis Program at the University of Washington.

The state programs and the National Health Policy Forum coordinate some of their activities, sharing research, for example, said Pamela Dickson, the Foundation's program officer for the state programs and, before she joined the Foundation staff, an assistant health commissioner for New Jersey. The national Forum reports that it has assisted the state-based forums when they have asked for information or contacts and has provided them with copies of its Issue Briefs and site visit reports.

*Sources: Forums on Health Care Issues for New Jersey Policymakers.* Grant Results Report, The Robert Wood Johnson Foundation. (www.rwjf.org/reports/grr/023538s. htm); *Feasibility Study of Replicating the New Jersey Capitol Forums on Health and Medical Care.* Grant Results Brief, The Robert Wood Johnson Foundation. (www.rwjf. org/reports/grr/029577.htm); *Annual Progress Report.* National Health Policy Forum, 2000, p. 12.

# Notes

1. National Health Policy Forum's Web site (www.nhpf.org).
2. *Proposal to The Robert Wood Johnson Foundation for a Renewal of Its Grant.* National Health Policy Forum, June 1999.
3. Ibid.
4. Ibid.
5. Gencarelli, D. M. *Average Wholesale Price for Prescription Drugs: Is There a More Appropriate Pricing Mechanism?* Issue Brief, no. 775. National Health Policy Forum, June 7, 2002, p. 14.
6. Super, N. *Medigap: Prevalence, Premiums, and Opportunities for Reform.* Issue Brief, no. 782. National Health Policy Forum, Sept. 9, 2002, p. 20.
7. Salinsky, E. *Will the Nation Be Ready for the Next Bioterrorism Attack? Mending Gaps in the Public Health Infrastructure.* Issue Brief, no. 776. National Health Policy Forum, June 12, 2002, p. 17.
8. *Proposal to The Robert Wood Johnson Foundation . . .* (1999), pp. 5–6.
9. *Annual Progress Report,* National Health Policy Forum, 1998, p. 3.
10. *Annual Progress Report,* National Health Policy Forum, 2000, p. 9.
11. For a short history of the dispute, see Nichols, L. M., and Reischauer, R. D. "Who Really Wants Price Competition in Medicare Managed Care?" *Health Affairs,* 2000, *19,* 30–43.
12. *Annual Progress Report* (2000), p. 9.

# Vulnerable Populations Portfolio

# 8

# The Injury Free Coalition for Kids

*Paul Brodeur*

---

## Editors' Introduction

Beginning in 1988, The Robert Wood Johnson Foundation supported a series of programs focused on reducing injuries to children living in low-income neighborhoods. The idea for the initial program came from two Harlem Hospital physicians who treated injured children from the gritty inner-city area of New York City surrounding the hospital and who carried out research on children's injuries. Disturbed by the number of children who came to the emergency room with injuries from gunshot wounds, traffic accidents, falls from windows, and the like, the physicians approached The Robert Wood Johnson Foundation about funding a pilot program designed to prevent injuries to children. The Foundation was receptive to the idea and made an award for what became the Harlem Hospital Injury Prevention Program.

The story of this program and its successor, the nationwide Injury Free Coalition for Kids program, is told by Paul Brodeur, a former staff writer at the *New Yorker* and a frequent contributor to The Robert Wood Johnson Foundation

*Anthology.* It illustrates how the Foundation sometimes works in addressing serious health issues: taking promising ideas suggested by knowledgeable outsiders, testing them on a relatively small scale, expanding the test on a larger scale, and then funding those same experienced individuals to assist those who are newer to the field.

Supporting efforts to reduce childhood injuries is a logical component of The Robert Wood Johnson Foundation's long-standing interest in improving children's health, which is woven into almost every area of its grantmaking. In the 2001 volume of the *Anthology,* Sharon Begley and Ruby Hearn wrote that between 1972 and 2001 the Foundation had made more than two thousand grants totaling $860 million to improve children's health.[1] Since then, the Foundation has awarded an additional $388 million.

The Harlem Hospital Injury Prevention Program foreshadowed the expansion of the Foundation's grantmaking to include health as well as health care. When the program was initially funded, most Foundation grants were directed toward improving the medical care system. In contrast, the injury prevention initiative was a classic prevention program—one that attempted to get at some of the causes of poor health, such as unsafe playgrounds and traffic accidents. Under a reorganization of the Foundation that occurred in 1998, improving health per se—for example, by reducing unhealthy behaviors such as smoking, drinking, and using illicit drugs, or by reducing preventable injuries—was given equal priority to improving health care.

1. Begley, S., and Hearn, R. P. "Children's Health Initiatives." In *To Improve Health and Health Care 2001: The Robert Wood Johnson Foundation Anthology.* San Francisco: Jossey-Bass, 2001.

—ɯ— I n the United States preventable injuries are the leading cause
of death for children from ages one to fourteen, accounting for more
deaths than cancer, AIDS, pneumonia, and all other diseases combined.
More than 5,000 children die each year of preventable injuries,[1] and nearly 40,000 are treated every day in hospital emergency rooms or doctors'
offices for broken bones, lacerations, burns, or other more serious injuries.[2]
Childhood injuries occur in a wide range of circumstances:

- *Motor vehicle injuries.* Among children between the ages
  of one and fourteen, motor vehicle injuries are the leading
  cause of death and hospitalization. Every ninety seconds,
  a child is killed or injured while riding in an automobile or
  a truck. In 1999 (the latest year for which fatality data were
  available at the time of this writing), more than 2,000 children under sixteen were killed in car crashes, and more than
  320,000 were injured. Nearly half of the children five and
  younger who were killed in car crashes were riding unre-
  strained by car safety seats, booster seats, or seat belts.
  Only about 6 percent of children aged four to eight ride in
  booster seats, the recommended safety seat for this group.[3]

- *Drowning.* Drowning is the second leading cause of injury-
  related death among children between the ages of one and
  fourteen. Some 1,000 children drown each year in the
  United States, most of them in backyard swimming pools.
  For every child who drowns, 4 others are hospitalized, and
  15 receive emergency care for near-drowning.[4]

- *Fires.* Fires are the third leading cause of injury-related
  deaths among children up to the age of nine. Children
  under four are at greatest risk for dying as a result of a residential fire. Ninety-five percent of scalds from hot liquids—
  the most frequent cause of nonfatal, nonfire injuries—occur
  among children younger than five.[5]

- *Bicycle crashes.* In 1999, 750 bicyclists died in crashes. More
  than one-quarter were children between the ages of five and

fifteen. And 140,000 children are treated each year in emergency rooms for head injuries sustained while the victims were bicycling. Only about 1 in 4 children between the ages of five and fourteen wear helmets when riding bicycles.[6]

- *Falls.* Falls are the leading cause of visits to emergency rooms by children, accounting for as many as 3 million visits a year. More than 40 percent of these falls occur among infants, toddlers, and preschoolers.[7]

- *Pedestrian injuries.* In 1999, some 600 child pedestrians fifteen and younger died from traffic-related injuries. And 27,000 sustained nonfatal injuries.[8]

- *Playground injuries.* More than 200,000 children fourteen and younger are treated annually in emergency rooms for playground-related injuries. More than a third of the injuries sustained on playgrounds are severe—including fractures, internal injuries, and concussions. Most playground injuries are associated with the use of climbing equipment, slides, and swings. Almost 70 percent of the injuries involving playground equipment occur on public playgrounds.[9]

- *Poison.* In 1999, poison control centers in the United States reported more than 2 million exposures to poison. More than half of these occurred among children younger than six.[10]

In large part, the distressing situation highlighted by these statistics can be explained by the fact that, until recently, few communities and pediatric trauma centers had undertaken significant efforts to reduce the incidence of unintentional injuries being sustained by children—particularly those living in crowded urban areas. Instead of acting to prevent childhood injuries, most pediatric trauma centers have merely treated injuries, viewing them as accidental and, as such, random, unexpected, and not preventable. Only within the past fifteen years has there been a major effort to reverse this reactive attitude and to engage in a proactive, preventive approach to the problem of childhood injury. The new initiative has focused on studying where, why, when, and how childhood injuries occur, and then devising programs and interventions designed to reduce their incidence.

## —w— Early Efforts to Prevent Childhood Injuries

The effort to chronicle and prevent childhood injuries has its genesis in the vision and determination of a single person—in this case, Barbara Barlow, who became chief of pediatric surgery at the Harlem Hospital Center in New York City in 1975. What Dr. Barlow encountered during her early months at the Harlem Hospital Center, a public hospital affiliated with the College of Physicians and Surgeons at Columbia University, led her to suspect that Harlem and other parts of northern Manhattan were experiencing an extraordinarily increased incidence of childhood injury compared with the rest of New York City. "I had never seen anything like it at any of the other hospitals with which I had been associated," she said not long ago. "Dozens upon dozens of children were being brought in who had fallen out of windows, been hit by cars, been hurt on playgrounds, or been shot, stabbed, or assaulted by other means. Since the predominant weight of a small child is in the head, children who were falling from high windows were falling headfirst, with catastrophic results. In fact, more than one in four of them were dying."

In 1972, the New York City Health Department had developed a pilot program to prevent window falls, after a study conducted between 1965 and 1969 showed that falls from heights during this period had caused 12 percent of all deaths among children under fifteen years of age, with 123 deaths (82 percent) occurring as a result of window falls. The program, which was called "Children Can't Fly," included door-to-door visits by outreach workers, who counseled parents on preventive measures and distributed free window guards. Between 1973 and 1975, the number of deaths among New York City children caused by falls from heights decreased by 35 percent, but the problem remained severe. In 1974 and 1975—a period in which thirty-two thousand free window guards were distributed to some 8,400 families—170 children who had fallen from windows were admitted to city hospitals for treatment of injuries that included skull fractures, brain damage, paralysis, ruptured spleens, loss of eyesight, and other incapacitating trauma.

In 1976, the New York City Board of Health passed a law requiring owners of multiple dwellings to provide window guards for apartments in which children ten or younger were residing. The law stipulated that all landlords be in compliance by the end of March 1979.[11] At that time Dr. Barlow, who had already established a pediatric trauma registry at the Harlem Hospital Center, began working with the director of the school health program to educate the parents of young children in Harlem about the importance of informing landlords of the requirement to install window guards. Within two years there was a 96 percent reduction in the number of children falling out of windows in central Harlem.[12]

"The success of the window guard program convinced me not only that other urban communities should establish similar initiatives but also that urban public hospitals might be able to play a leadership role in preventing childhood deaths and injuries from other causes," Barlow has said.

In 1982, Barlow and some colleagues from the College of Physicians and Surgeons of Columbia University published a paper in the *Journal of Pediatric Surgery* in which they wrote that during the previous ten years, 108 children sixteen years of age and under had been admitted to the Pediatric Surgical Service of Harlem Hospital with gunshot wounds. Half of them had been shot by guns held by other children. More than 1 in 20 of them had died. Since only one child had been admitted to the Pediatric Surgical Service for treatment of gunshot wounds during the ten years preceding the review period, it was obvious that gunshot wounds had become a significant new source of mortality and morbidity among children living in Harlem. In their paper Barlow and her colleagues pointed out that one obvious reason for the increase was the ease with which it had become possible to obtain handguns in Harlem. They also pointed out a second, less obvious reason—the so-called 1973 Rockefeller Drug Laws (named after Governor Nelson Rockefeller), which imposed very stiff penalties on adults convicted of drug possession.

As a result of the 1973 law, drug dealers in Harlem began recruiting children from twelve to sixteen years of age to sell drugs on the street. The dealers armed the children with handguns to intimidate rivals and enforce the drug-selling code of behavior, knowing that drug possession, drug selling, and gun possession among youngsters of their age were handled by family court and were usually punished by probation or short-term incarceration in a juvenile home. Since most drug-dealing children were school dropouts, Barlow and her colleagues in the Pediatric Surgical Service worked closely with the hospital's Social Service Department and its Division of Child Psychiatry to evaluate children who had been admitted for gunshot wounds, encourage them to return to school, and support them in changing their dangerous lifestyle. In their paper in the *Journal of Pediatric Surgery,* she and her coauthors acknowledged that such efforts were not uniformly successful but declared that "we do have many former patients back in school, attending technical schools or colleges— heading toward productive lives."[13]

Meanwhile, Barlow had been sending grant proposals to various federal minority health programs and other governmental agencies, asking for financial support for a program to prevent childhood injuries. It was a futile and discouraging process. "Whenever and wherever I put in for a grant, I was told that the problem of childhood injuries was insoluble because such injuries were the result of accidents, and accidents were bound to happen and were thus unpreventable," she recalls, bristling at the memory. A white-haired, brown-eyed, gentle-faced woman in her middle sixties, she has a will of iron when it comes to preventing childhood injuries, and zero tolerance for ascribing them to accidents. Indeed, for Barlow there is no such thing as a childhood accident. There are only preventable childhood injuries.

Between January 1983 and December 1987, Barlow and some colleagues—among them Maureen Durkin, associate professor of clinical epidemiology at Columbia University's School of Public Health and Sergievsky Center; Leslie Davidson of Columbia University's College of Physicians and Surgeons; and Margaret Heagarty, head of the Department of Pediatrics at the Harlem Hospital Center—undertook an epidemiological study of the occurrence of severe injuries among the eighty-nine thousand children under the age of seventeen who were living in northern Manhattan. The study was the first ever conducted in the United States to assess the incidence of injury among inner-city children. Data collected on 2,761 injuries severe enough to require hospitalization and on eighty-three deaths during the five-year period showed Barlow's early hunch to have been correct. The rate for injuries causing hospitalization and death in northern Manhattan was significantly higher than in other parts of New York City and the nation. Indeed, the injury rate in central Harlem was nearly twice that of the United States. Falls accounted for the highest incidence of injury, followed by vehicle-related injuries (two-thirds of them to pedestrians and nearly a quarter to bicycle riders), toxic and medical ingestions, burns, assaults, and gunshot wounds. Assaults caused nearly one in ten injury hospitalizations and more than one in three injury deaths. Gunshot wounds were the leading cause of injury mortality, accounting for 14 percent of the deaths.[14]

Even though the data clearly showed the necessity of undertaking preventive measures to reduce the number of childhood injuries in northern Manhattan, Barlow continued to be stymied in her efforts to gain financial support. The turning point came in late 1987, when Barlow's colleague Margaret Heagarty, who had been a Robert Wood Johnson Health Policy Fellow, approached Ruby Hearn, a senior vice president at the Foundation, and suggested that since the Foundation was working to improve the health of children, it ought to consider giving a small grant to help prevent childhood injuries. Hearn then sent Michael Beachler, a young program officer who had joined the Foundation six months earlier, to meet with Barlow, Heagarty, and Durkin at Harlem Hospital, with the idea of determining whether an injury prevention program might be viable.

"We sat around a table and floated a bunch of ideas," Beachler recalls. "The thing that stood out was Dr. Barlow's passion and commitment. Within a week or two she had sent me the results of the northern Manhattan study, as well as a concept paper outlining some specific interventions that could be taken to reduce the incidence of childhood injuries. During the next few months, we worked together to frame a proposal for a small program designed to form a coalition between Harlem Hospital's Departments of Pediatrics and Pediatric Surgery and various city and community agencies, in order to continue the window safety initiative, improve playground safety, and develop new projects designed to reduce injury to children in central Harlem."

In 1988, the Foundation awarded Harlem Hospital the first of two grants (totaling $541,000 over four years) to enable Barlow and her colleagues to develop a pilot injury prevention program for children living in central Harlem.

## —ᴍᴍ— The Harlem Hospital Injury Prevention Program

The Harlem Hospital Injury Prevention Program, which grew out of this grant, became one of the most successful ad hoc projects in the history of The Robert Wood Johnson Foundation. Under Barlow's direction the new project hit the ground running. Hypothesizing that motor vehicle pedestrian injuries would decrease if children stopped using the streets as play areas, she and program staff members surveyed and photographed several dozen parks, playgrounds, and schoolyards in central Harlem to document unsafe conditions—among them dangerous equipment, unpadded surfaces, rodent infestation, and drug dealing. During the next ten years, they worked with the New York City Board of Education and local schools to build fifty-five new playgrounds at public schools and day-care centers, and with the New York City Department of Parks and Recreation to rebuild playgrounds in eleven parks, equipping them with soft safety surfaces and rubber swings. Child pedestrian injuries dropped during 1989, the first year of the initiative, and not a single child was admitted to Harlem Hospital in 1991 for a swing injury, which had previously been the major cause of equipment-related park and playground injuries.

Working with the New York City Department of Transportation, coalition members instituted an intensive pedestrian and bicycle safety program for grammar school children, undertook to provide more than five hundred bicycle helmets free or at cost, repaired children's bicycles, and formed an Urban Bike Corps. In collaboration with the New York Emergency Medical Services, they established a "Kids, Injuries, and Street Smarts" curriculum on how to deal with violence-related situations. With the help of the Central Harlem Board of Education, they initiated a "No Guns in School" curriculum. Together with the Department of Parks, they developed a "Greening of Harlem" program that taught children horticulture and encouraged them to plant and care for school playground gardens.

With the support of private and corporate donors, they continued the window guard campaign and developed a burn prevention curriculum that included the distribution of smoke detectors. They also started a variety of programs to involve children in the hours they were not in school—when injuries were most likely to occur. These included a hospital-based art studio with more than two hundred participants, a hospital-based dance clinic involving several hundred girls, a program in which more than one hundred children were encouraged to paint murals, a Harlem Little League with twenty-four teams, a soccer league, and a winter baseball clinic. A Safe Kids/Healthy Neighborhoods Coalition provided education in teen pregnancy prevention, gun safety for parents, and alternatives to violence for adolescents and adults.

During 1989, major injury admissions to Harlem Hospital's Pediatric Trauma Service dropped 14 percent—the first recorded decrease since 1975. By the end of 1992, when funding from The Robert Wood Johnson Foundation ended, there had been a 41 percent decrease in major trauma hospital admissions for children living in central Harlem, as compared with admissions during the 1983–1987 period. There was also a 50 percent decrease in motor vehicle pedestrian injuries, a 50 percent drop in bicycle injuries, and a 50 percent drop in serious playground injuries. In addition, a 50 percent decrease in assault and gun injuries among Harlem adolescents had been recorded.[15]

By this time, the Injury Prevention Program had received considerable media attention and had been able to raise more than $1 million in additional financial resources. The program had also begun to serve as a model for injury prevention projects that were being planned at city, state, and national levels. The New York State Health Department's injury prevention people had expressed interest in replicating it in problem areas within their jurisdiction; and Harlem Hospital's injury prevention resource book had been circulated to ten groups across the nation whose members had requested help in setting up similar projects.

## —⚬⚬— Expanding the Injury Prevention Program

The dramatic reduction in injuries sustained by children living in central Harlem between 1988 and 1992 went a long way toward persuading staff members at The Robert Wood Johnson Foundation, who had been skeptical initially, that the Injury Prevention Program had been worth funding and that similar initiatives in other inner-city communities might also warrant support. In 1994, Foundation program officer Michael Beachler approached Barbara Barlow about an initiative that would expand the program by disseminating it as a model to hospital-based sites in other metropolitan areas. As a result, Harlem Hospital received a three-year grant of $1 million to continue its injury prevention program and to use it as a model in pediatric trauma centers in five cities with high childhood injury rates. The replication sites included Allegheny General Hospital in Pittsburgh; Children's Memorial Hospital in Chicago; Hughes Spalding Children's Hospital in Atlanta; Children's Mercy Hospital in Kansas City, Missouri; and the Harbor-UCLA Medical Center in Torrance, California. Interest earned on the Foundation's grant to Harlem Hospital provided half of the funding for a sixth site at St. Louis Children's Hospital, and to extend the program for an additional six months in Pittsburgh, Chicago, and Kansas City.

To accelerate the formation of injury control programs at the replication sites, members of the Harlem Hospital Injury Prevention Program provided technical assistance for all aspects of the model, including community outreach, coalition building, safe play space design, safe activities, safety education, and evaluation of program effectiveness. The latter proved especially difficult, because each site had unique problems with data collection, ranging from a lack of hospital, city, and state databases, to poorly coded hospital data, state data collected without zip code information, and the refusal of some medical examiners to release data on injury deaths. However, by the summer of 1998, when funding ended for the first phase of the program, all of the hospital sites either had injury surveillance systems that were in operation or systems that were being set up. At that time the Harlem Hospital Injury Prevention Program and the six replication programs were given a new name—the Injury Free Coalition for Kids.[16]

### The Injury Free Coalition for Kids of Kansas City

Although Harlem Hospital's Injury Prevention Program provided a blueprint, each expansion site developed its own response to childhood injury. Children's Mercy Hospital, in Kansas City, Missouri, for example, serves 135 counties in western Missouri and eastern Kansas. Initial injury surveillance data and research showed a high rate of injury among children in Kansas City from gunshot wounds and motor vehicle crashes. Play-ground injuries also resulted in many childhood visits to the emergency room. In partnership with Kansas City officials, the police department, and local residents, the Injury Free Coalition at Children's Mercy devel-oped a program called "Safe Zones," which concentrated on building safe playgrounds for children in neighborhoods with the highest injury rates. Among other programs established by the Kansas City coalition were psy-chological counseling for children who witness violence, a Safe Kids Safe Homes program, bike-riding safety clinics and bike rodeos, training in the wearing of bike helmets, a teen drama club, toy safety, playground safe-ty, fireworks safety, and airbag safety. In partnership with the Kansas City Royals baseball team, the hospital also provided Safe-at-Home Boxes con-taining safety items such as electrical outlet covers, medicine cabinet latches, poison control information, and home safety checklists.

### The Injury Free Coalition for Kids of Atlanta

The Hughes Spalding Children's Hospital provides health care to the neighborhoods and communities of Atlanta, including Grady Homes, a 495-unit low-income housing project in which many young children re-side. Injury data collected on children living in the project showed that many of them—especially younger children—were being hurt in their homes as a result of falls and poisoning. Door-to-door surveys conducted by Injury Free Coalition personnel revealed that safety gates were used by fewer than one-third of the families with young children; that about one-third of the children under one year of age were using walkers in spite of their danger; and that nearly one-third of all families stored hazardous household products in unlocked areas accessible to small children. How-ever, when coalition members visited residents in Grady Homes to look for unsafe conditions, they were greeted with suspicion, as outsiders. As a result, the coalition changed its strategy and built a life-size three-room house on wheels, called "Safety House," which contained a kitchen, a bathroom, and a baby's bedroom. By showing Safety House to the resi-dents of Grady Homes and other low-income communities, the coalition was able to demonstrate unsafe conditions and remedies for them in a way that proved to be nonthreatening and productive. Among other programs initiated by Injury Free Atlanta were car seat programs for infants and young children, bike safety rodeos and bike helmet giveaways, safe Halloween training, burn and poison prevention, and playground safety.

### The Injury Free Coalition for Kids of St. Louis

The Injury Prevention Coalition at St. Louis Children's Hospital concentrated its efforts on the Hamilton Heights area, a community of 5,500 residents with many children living in single-family households, a median annual household income of $16,000, and serious problems with drugs and gangs. Among the coalition's interventions to deal with these problems were the Cease Fire for the Holidays appeal, the Gun Safety Poster contest, the Toy Gun Buyback for Books, the Community Violence Lecture, and the Pediatric Trauma Workshop on Gun Wounds.

Early data showed that African American children living in Missouri were suffering twice the rate of burn injury as white children and that the highest rate was occurring among African American boys who lived in metropolitan counties. Using the zip codes of young burn victims who visited the emergency room at Children's Hospital or were admitted to the hospital, members of the St. Louis Injury Prevention Coalition were able to identify neighborhoods with the highest number of burn injuries. At that point, working with the St. Louis Fire Department, they visited those neighborhoods and installed smoke detectors in several hundred homes that lacked them. In addition, they trained children and adult residents in fire safety awareness. By 2001, there was a steep reduction in the number of pediatric burns being treated at St. Louis Children's Hospital, although how much of this decrease can be attributed to the coalition's initiatives cannot be known with certainty.[17]

### The Injury Free Coalitions for Kids of Pittsburgh and Worcester

The earliest and one of the most successful replication programs was begun in 1994 at Allegheny General Hospital in Pittsburgh by Michael

Hirsh, a pediatric surgeon, who pioneered a number of innovative projects at Allegheny General before moving to Mercy Hospital of Pittsburgh and establishing a second replication program there. "Soon after we started up in 1994, we learned that gunshot wounds were the leading cause of childhood injury among children between the ages of five and nineteen in Allegheny County," he recalled not long ago. "We also learned that we had a very negative image in the community. At a neighborhood meeting attended by then attorney general Janet Reno, people not only were bitterly critical of the hospital but also were convinced that it was profiting from the injuries occurring to their children instead of working to prevent them. As for the kids, when asked what their perception of a hospital was, they would often as not reply 'a place I go when I get shot.'"

Hirsh, who now heads the Injury Free Coalition at the UMass Memorial Children's Medical Center in Worcester, Massachusetts, went on to say that the Pittsburgh Police Department had operated a gun return program since 1990, but because people had to turn in their weapons at precinct stations, where there were surveillance cameras, the police had managed to collect only about twenty-five guns. "Some years earlier I had heard about a carpet store owner in Washington Heights (New York City) who offered free carpets in return for guns," he said. "With that in mind, we started a Goods for Guns program under the slogan 'Guns and Kids Don't Mix,' offering $25 for a rifle or long gun, and $50 for a handgun, in the form of department store gift certificates. On the morning of the first day, the line of people waiting to turn in weapons was three blocks long. We ran out of certificates in an hour, so we went to the nearest ATM machine, and, after depleting our personal stock of cash, ended up handing out vouchers. During the first two Saturdays of September, we collected 1,400 guns. During the past nine years, the program has collected 7,800 guns—more than any other buyback program in the country—at a total cost of about $435,000. That, by the way, is approximately the cost of one spinal cord injury to a child."

Seeking to prevent motor vehicle injuries to children, Hirsh and his colleagues at Injury Free Pittsburgh used funds from The Robert Wood Johnson Foundation and other private foundations and corporations to design and build a life-size model city street, called "Safety Street," which is on permanent display in a parking lot at the Pittsburgh Children's Museum. The model contains stores, traffic signals, cars, bicycles, a school bus, and recordings of city street noise. It is visited each year by thirty thousand city and suburban schoolchildren, who learn valuable lessons about how to make safe choices when crossing a street, riding a bike, or exiting from a school bus.

In order to counter the peer pressure that encourages children to drop out of school and join gangs, Hirsh and his colleagues established Health Rangers—a mentoring program that gives middle school children the opportunity to develop one-on-one relationships with adult role models. The program, which began in 1994, selected marginal kids—those who exhibited promise but were considered at risk for future trouble—and paired them with hospital mentors in order to increase their self-esteem, broaden their outlook, and provide them with information about possible careers. "We were careful not to limit our mentors to doctors and nurses, because we didn't want to set the bar too high and scare the kids away," Hirsh said. "So we also recruited cooks, dieticians, housekeepers, security guards, van drivers, and helicopter pilots. The program started with twenty-five seventh graders. The program has since grown to include seven middle schools and three additional hospitals, and has resulted in improved school attendance and academic performance among children who have been enrolled in it."

## —〰— Further Expansion of the Injury Free Coalition for Kids

In July 1998, The Robert Wood Johnson Foundation approved a new $3.1 million grant for the development over a three-year period of a strengthened network of pediatric injury centers, as well as the establishment of a technical assistance resource center on hospital-based pediatric injury prevention. Under the direction of Barbara Barlow, the network and the center were to work with the expansion sites to help them become institutionalized in their hospitals and to further develop their programs.

## *The Injury Prevention Coalition for Kids of Philadelphia*

Using funds from the grant, TraumaLink—the center for injury prevention research of the Children's Hospital of Philadelphia—joined the network. At about the same time, with consultation and guidance from the Injury Free Coalition resource center, the Children's Medical Center of Dallas created an injury prevention program that was self-funded.

Like other injury prevention sites, the ones in Philadelphia and Dallas had unique problems that demanded special interventions. West Philadelphia—the immediate service area of the Children's Hospital of Philadelphia—is home to more than sixty thousand children under the age of eighteen. Nearly half of them live in single-parent, female-headed households, and 26 percent of these households exist below the poverty level. Between 1997 and 1999, members of the Injury Free Coalition for Kids of Philadelphia identified the leading causes of childhood injury. They found that in West Philadelphia approximately 40 percent of children who were severely injured or admitted to the hospital had been hurt at home. Pedestrian and biking injuries also ranked high as causes for emergency room visits and hospitalization.

Using geographical mapping and community surveys, coalition staff members determined the locations of the most severe and prevalent home injuries, and then joined with the local SAFE KIDS coalition and other groups to train volunteers, who provided in-home safety education, home safety inspections, and home safety equipment, such as smoke detectors, safety gates, nightlights, and crib and cabinet latches.

Using TraumaLink's surveillance system, the Injury Free Coalition for Kids of Philadelphia collected information on the pre-injury behavior of children hit by cars. It showed that most of them had been playing in the street. The coalition then mapped the locations of child pedestrian injuries to identify patterns and troublesome locations, and, together with the city's Department of Recreation, began to develop structured activities for children who lived and played in the vicinity of trouble spots. In partnership with the Philadelphia Department of Public Health and the SAFE KIDS campaign, the coalition also mounted a broad effort to distribute helmets to children who had been identified as high-risk as a result of bicycle-related or similar injuries. As a result, more than four hundred Philadelphia children who were injured while riding bicycles or scooters or roller-blading received a safety helmet before going home.[18]

## The Injury Free Coalition for Kids of Dallas

In Dallas, where backyard swimming pools are common, members of the injury prevention program faced a different set of problems. According to statistics from the Texas Department of Health, ninety-five children died by drowning in the Dallas area between 1995 and 1998. The high rate of drowning was compounded by the fact that for every child who drowns, four other children nearly drown, and one in five of those who nearly drown are left with severe lifelong disabilities. Since the Injury Free Coalition for Kids of Dallas was a member of the Dallas County Child Death and Infant Mortality Review Team, which reviews the death of every child that occurs in Dallas, the coalition was able to determine that most drowning victims were toddlers or young children; that most drownings occurred in pools that were not fenced separately from the house; that many drownings occurred in apartment pools; and that most of the drownings were silent events, with children toppling quietly into pools without thrashing or crying out. To deal with the problem, the coalition developed a drowning prevention curriculum that included a slide presentation, video, and script, and presented it at a safety forum for health, safety, and community professionals. With the help of volunteers from the Texas Women's University School of Occupational Therapy, the coalition then took its drowning prevention message to the broader Dallas community. In addition, the coalition worked with the Texas Department of Health in seeking stronger laws to regulate fencing for semiprivate and private swimming pools.[19]

In July 2001, The Robert Wood Johnson Foundation authorized up to $15 million over a five-year period to extend the dissemination of the injury prevention program to forty hospitals that had pediatric trauma centers and were interested in replicating the model. Under the new initiative each additional hospital site would receive a grant of $50,000 a year for three, four, or five years. By the end of 2002, the network of injury prevention sites had reached twenty-seven, with thirteen additional sites planned for 2003.[20]

The Foundation's $15 million grant also provided for the establishment of a National Program Office for the Injury Free Coalition, which was set up in 2002 under the direction of Dr. Barlow within the Department of Epidemiology of Columbia University's Mailman School of Public Health. The National Program Office provides the program's injury prevention sites with brochures and safety checklists and an array of home safety devices—among them smoke alarms, bath thermometers, window safety disks, choke tubes for measuring small items that children might swallow, and cabinet door locks. It also coordinates research activities across sites and provides technical assistance by conducting workshops, helping to calculate population-based injury rates, and obtaining injury information from state agencies charged with maintaining statewide hospital discharge data.

## —⚍— A Closer Look: Visits to Three of the Coalitions

A closer look at three coalitions—those of Miami, San Diego, and Chicago—illustrates how the Injury Free Coalition for Kids program has developed.

### *The Injury Free Coalition for Kids of Miami*

One of the new kids on the block is the Injury Free Coalition for Kids of Miami, which started up in April 2001 at the University of Miami Department of Pediatrics Mailman Center for Child Development, with support from Jackson Memorial Hospital. The coalition is directed by Dr. Judy Schaechter, an assistant professor of pediatrics, who, like many of her colleagues, is passionate about the necessity of preventing childhood injuries. "Miami is the poorest large city in the nation, and it leads the nation in violent crime," Schaechter said. "When I joined the Department of Pediatrics, in 1996, there were more admissions to Jackson Memorial Hospital and the Ryder Trauma Center for childhood injuries caused by violence than for injuries caused by motor vehicle crashes. Why, we were treating thirteen- and fourteen-year-olds practically every day for gunshot wounds! Between 1994 and 1998, gunshot wounds caused 123 deaths among Miami children. Half of them were killed in their own homes, or in the home of a relative or friend—places where they should have been the most safe. Nearly half of the children under twelve years of age who were the victims of fatal violence were killed by their mother's intimate partner. Most of the weapons involved in these shootings were owned by parents, a family member, or a friend of the family. I call them household guns."

Schaechter went on to say that in 1999 she started a coalition against violence called "Not One More," with the aid of a $7,500 grant from the American Academy of Pediatrics. "The name was intended to stand as a declaration by the community that not one more child should die by violence," she explained. "In October of 2000, supporters of Not One More developed the Partnership for the Study and Prevention of Violence, which later became the lead agency for the Injury Free Coalition for Kids of Miami. Teaming up with Miami-Dade County mayor Alex Penelas, school board members, community organizations, business leaders, and the police, the Partnership and Not One More passed out brochures against violence, distributed more than five hundred gun locks, produced a gun lock video with the assistance of the Miami-Dade Police Department, and initiated a guns-for-gifts exchange program that netted nearly 450 handguns and rifles. That same year, in conjunction with law enforcement and health officials, the Partnership set up a violent injury statistics system, which now tracks fatal and nonfatal injuries caused by violence in the greater Miami area."

"In 2001," Schaechter continued, "with money from The Robert Wood Johnson Foundation and a matching grant from Miami-Dade County, we became a member of the nationwide Injury Free Coalition for Kids and were able to set up a program called InReach, which works closely with community residents to support solutions to the problem posed by violence. InReach also develops projects encouraging youth activities, such as talent shows, musical instrument lessons, and participation in sports. Adult mentoring activities include swimming lessons, football clinics, and projects for improving the environment. All told, we have two hundred kids enrolled in ten programs."

### The Injury Free Coalition for Kids of San Diego

An even newer kid on the block is the Injury Free Coalition for Kids of San Diego. It started up in March 2002 and operates in partnership with the San Diego Safe Kids Coalition and the Center for Healthier Communities at the Children's Hospital and Health Center, about three miles northeast of downtown San Diego. The Center for Healthier Communities was launched in 1996 and serves as the lead agency of the Injury Free Coalition. As is the case in other cities, unintentional injuries are the leading cause of death for San Diego children, with motor vehicle collisions being the leading cause of death and severe injury among children five to fourteen years of age. Statistics gathered by the Safe Kids Coalition show that a vast majority of child safety seats in San Diego are incorrectly installed. Indeed, the misuse rate has been estimated to be more than 85 percent. To combat this problem, the Center for Healthier Communities, the Safe Kids Coalition, the Injury Free Coalition for Kids of San Diego, and partner organizations have conducted more than one thousand child safety seat inspections and prepared an up-to-date child safety seat handout that includes compliance with 2002 California state regulations.

Pedestrian injuries are the second leading cause of unintentional injuries among San Diego children. Data gathered in 1999 revealed that Mid-City—a heavily Hispanic and new immigrant neighborhood—had a far greater proportion of child pedestrian injuries than the rest of San Diego County. In fact, although Mid-City children under the age of fifteen accounted for less than 7 percent of the total population of the county, they sustained 16 percent of the pedestrian injuries in the county.[21] In 2000, with a small grant from the University of California, San Francisco, and the California Department of Health Services, Children's Hospital and Health Center and a large number of community partners implemented the Safe Routes to School project in Mid-City. To begin with, three schools with a high incidence of childhood pedestrian injury were identified through Trauma Registry data, police reports, and anecdotal information provided by parents and the members of neighborhood associations. Over the next two years, engineers from the California Institute of Traffic Safety analyzed traffic and pedestrian behavior at these locations and recommended specific remedies, such as the construction of new crosswalks, traffic signals, flashing "Don't Walk" signs, and footprint trails on sidewalks to guide young children to safe street-crossing points.

Since the spring of 2002, the Injury Free Coalition for Kids of San Diego and the Center for Healthier Communities have been in the process of expanding the Safe Routes to School project to southeast San Diego, a densely populated neighborhood that includes residents with Hispanic and African American backgrounds as well as many recent immigrants from Eritrea, Somalia, Ethiopia, Vietnam, and Cambodia. According to Cheri Fidler, the director of the Center for Healthier Communities, the cultural experience of many of the residents of southeast San Diego has not equipped them to cope with the pedestrian hazards of a large modern city. "I have been given to understand that people who have grown up in Mexico often teach their children to cross the street in the middle of a block rather than at a corner because corners are known to be the most dangerous place to cross a street in Mexico," she told a visitor to the Injury Free Coalition of San Diego's offices at the Euclid Health Center, in the southeast section of the city. "Other people have never driven cars and so are without any reference point that provides them with an awareness of how fast cars travel. Their children are especially at risk because children perceive, think about, and react to traffic differently from the way adults do."

### The Injury Free Coalition for Kids of Chicago

The Injury Free Coalition for Kids of Chicago functioned from the start in partnership with Children's Memorial Hospital of Chicago and the hospital-based Cabrini Green Youth Program (now called Chicago Youth Programs), an organization founded back in 1984 by medical students at Northwestern University to help children in Cabrini Green, a low-income housing project known for gang violence. One of the founders, Joseph

DiCara, went on to win a Robert Wood Johnson Community Health Leadership Award in 1998.

Like the five other original replication sites that were financed by The Robert Wood Johnson Foundation in the middle 1990s, the Injury Free Coalition for Kids of Chicago has developed a large number of programs and interventions as well as an extensive network of partnerships. The coalition is directed by Karen Sheehan, who is a pediatrician at Children's Memorial Hospital and an assistant professor of pediatrics at Northwestern University's Feinberg School of Medicine. She is also the medical director of the Chicago Youth Programs/Children's Memorial Clinic, where doctors and medical students not only provide care for inner-city children but also play in the gym with them, tutor them, and take them on field trips.

A longtime advocate of preventing childhood injuries, Sheehan joined the Cabrini Green Youth Program when she began her studies at Northwestern University's Medical School in 1984. "In those days, we paid for our big-brother-big-sister programs by passing around the hat in classroom," she recalls. "We've come a long way since then, but especially since 1995, when the Injury Free Coalition for Kids of Chicago began its partnership with Chicago Youth Programs and Children's Memorial Hospital."

"In 1995," Dr. Sheehan explained, "with funding from Bally Total Fitness, the coalition built a new playground in Cabrini Green. Last year, with the cooperation of Chicago Public Schools, the Chicago Park District, and a civic organization called 'Friends of the Parks,' we were able to refurbish half a dozen playgrounds in several other inner-city neighborhoods we serve. One of them is Washington Park, a neighborhood on the south side of Chicago, which ranks near the bottom of the city's communities in household income, employment, and school graduation, and near the top in terms of teen births and homicides. The other is the Uptown community, an ethnically diverse neighborhood that is populated by African Americans, Mexicans, Cambodians, and Vietnamese, and in which fifty-seven languages are spoken. Together with Children's Memorial Hospital, we have initiated a collaboration to expand injury free programs with the University of Chicago Children's Hospital, Stroger Hospital, the Rehabilitation Institute of Chicago, and Northwest Community Hospital in Arlington Heights. Recently, one of our former volunteers spearheaded a campaign to build our own headquarters building. It is now being constructed in Washington Park on land provided by the city, and it will house office space, a day-care center, and a basketball court."

Sheehan went on to say that during the past two years five hundred Safe-at-Home boxes paid for by funds from the Allstate Foundation have been distributed by the Injury Free Coalition and its partners to Chicago families through local health clinics and parenting programs in Chicago Public Schools. "The Safe-at-Home boxes contain smoke detectors, outlet covers, poison control information, home safety checklists, and safety door latches. We have also initiated a major initiative to reduce childhood injuries caused by falls—especially window falls. Thanks to a comprehensive report issued in 2001 by the Child Health Data Lab of the Children's Memorial Institute for Education and Research, we learned that falls are the leading cause of hospitalization for Chicago children, accounting for almost 30 percent of all unintentional injury hospitalizations. We also found out that falls from windows account for the highest single rate of hospitalization for two- and three-year-olds. In fact, every spring and summer, two to three kids in Chicago are hospitalized each week because of injuries resulting from window falls. As a result, we have embarked upon a priority program called 'Stop the Falls.' It includes educating families about how to prevent window falls, limiting any opening in a window to no more than four inches, and encouraging the use of releasable window guards that are affordable and easy to install. Eventually, we're hoping to achieve the same kind of result that was achieved in New York City, where mandatory use of window guards in multiple-story buildings has reduced the number of window falls by 96 percent."

## —⁗— Conclusion

Many of Sheehan's colleagues join her in calculating that the injury surveillance systems in operation at the Injury Free Coalition replication sites will not be able to provide statistical proof of reduced childhood injuries for several years to come. However, the National Program Office is hoping to speed up the process by assisting the replication sites in assessing data gathered by injury surveillance systems. In the meantime, the programs and interventions that have been developed at virtually all of the sites furnish powerful reasons to believe that a significant reduction in the rate of childhood injury within many inner-city neighborhoods is under way. Some Injury Free Coalition members have expressed reservations that the organization may be expanding too rapidly and that with a total of forty sites expected to be in operation by the end of 2003, it may be difficult to avoid the pitfalls of bureaucracy and to retain the kind of focus, purpose, and cohesion that has characterized the organization to this point. However, the leadership of Barbara Barlow and the directors of the established sites, who will act as mentors to the directors and staff members of the thirteen new sites that will be added in 2003, should ensure the continuation of the Coalition's high standards. Indeed, Barlow's goal—the establishment of an injury prevention program at every one of the more than one hundred children's hospitals in the United States—has been endorsed by the National Association of Children's Hospitals and Related Institutions. In April 2002, with the aid of a grant from The Robert Wood Johnson Foundation, the Injury Free Coalition for Kids took a step toward this goal by holding a two-day conference at which four-member teams from thirty-five of the Association's hospitals received instruction in how to develop injury prevention programs similar to the ones currently in operation at the Coalition's twenty-seven hospital sites across the nation. Such an initiative parallels the Foundation's policy of financing projects whose value can be demonstrated and whose operations can be replicated and widely disseminated.

## Notes

1. *Injury Fact Book, 2001–2002.* National Center for Injury Prevention and Control, Nov. 2001, p. 30.
2. *Call for Proposals: Injury Free Coalition for Kids.* The Robert Wood Johnson Foundation, May 2002, p. 2.
3. *Injury Fact Book . . .* (2001), pp. 37–38, 58, 74.
4. Ibid., pp. 36, 117.
5. *Injury Research Agenda.* National Center for Injury Prevention and Control, June 2001, pp. 17, 24.
6. *Injury Fact Book . . .* (2001), pp. 50, 53.

7. *Injury Research Agenda* (2001), pp. 17, 22.

8. *Injury Fact Book . . .* (2001), p. 78.

9. Ibid., p. 82.

10. Ibid., p. 84.

11. Spiegel, C. N., and Lindaman, F. C. "Children Can't Fly." *American Journal of Pediatric Health,* 1977, *67*(12).

12. Barlow, B., Niemirska, M., Gandhi, R. P., and Leblanc, W. "Ten Years of Experience with Falls from a Height in Children." *Journal of Pediatric Surgery,* 1983, *18*(4).

13. Barlow, B., Niemirska, M., and Gandhi, R. P. "Ten Years' Experience with Pediatric Gunshot Wounds." *Journal of Pediatric Surgery,* 1982, *17*(6).

14. Davidson, L. L., and others. "The Epidemiology of Severe Injuries to Children in Northern Manhattan: Methods and Incidence Rates." *Pediatric and Perinatal Epidemiology,* 1992, 6, 153–156.

15. *Prevention of Injury to Children of Harlem, Final Report: Robert Wood Johnson Foundation Grant #13396.* College of Physicians and Surgeons of Columbia University, Aug. 1990, pp. 486–505; *Annual Progress Report: Year 1, Robert Wood Johnson Foundation Grant #14056.* College of Physicians and Surgeons of Columbia University, Aug. 1991, pp. 567–597; Davidson, L. L., and others. "The Impact of the Safe Kids/Healthy Neighborhoods Injury Prevention Program in Harlem, 1988 through 1991." *American Journal of Public Health,* 1994, *84*(4); Laraque, D., Barlow, B., Durkin, M., and Heagarty, M. "Injury Prevention in an Urban Setting: Challenges and Successes." *Bulletin of the New York Academy of Medicine,* Summer 1995.

16. *Dissemination of a Model Injury Prevention Program, Final Grant Report, #023514.* College of Physicians and Surgeons of Columbia University, July 1, 1998.

17. Quayle, K. S., and others. "Description of Missouri Children Who Suffer Burn Injuries." *Injury Prevention,* 2000, 6, 255–258.

18. *The Injury Free Coalition for Kids: A Passion for Prevention.* Special Report, The Robert Wood Johnson Foundation, Sept. 2000, pp. 15–17, 24.

19. Ibid., pp. 9–10.

20. The sites selected in 2001 were Children's Hospital of Pittsburgh; Cincinnati Children's Hospital Medical Center; UMass Memorial

Children's Medical Center in Worcester; Children's Hospital and Health Center in San Diego; Connecticut Children's Medical Center in Hartford; the University of Miami's Jackson Memorial Hospital; and Children's Hospital at Columbia University's Presbyterian Medical Center in New York City. The sites added in 2002 were the Harborview Medical Center and the Children's Hospital of Seattle; the Children's Hospital of Michigan in Detroit; the Hennepin County Medical Center in Minneapolis; the Pitt County Memorial Hospital in Greenville, North Carolina; the Arkansas Children's Hospital in Little Rock; the Rhode Island Hospital in Providence; Children's Hospital in Boston; Children's National Medical Center in Washington, D.C.; the University Health System in San Antonio, Texas; Johns Hopkins Children's Center in Baltimore; the University of Chicago Children's Memorial Hospital; and Children's Hospital of Austin in Texas.

21. Children's Hospital and Health Center, San Diego. "Pediatric Injuries." *Connections,* Jan.-Feb. 2001, p. 3.

# 9

# The Homeless Prenatal Program

*Digby Diehl*

## Editors' Introduction

In each issue of The Robert Wood Johnson Foundation *Anthology,* we present a close look at a single project representing a smaller than typical investment by the Foundation, in the hope that it will tell, in more intimate detail, the story of how the project evolved, who the players were that made it happen, and what general lessons can be derived from it. This chapter focuses on the Homeless Prenatal Program, a small nonprofit organization in San Francisco dedicated to working with pregnant women who are homeless.

It has received grants for three separate projects from the Foundation since 1992. Two came through the Local Initiative Funding Partners program, under which the Foundation offers matching grants to create partnerships with local foundations to support innovative, community-based projects helping underserved and vulnerable populations.[1] The Homeless Prenatal Program was one of a very few that were given two Local Initiative Funding Partners awards: the first for its work with homeless pregnant women and the second for its work providing services to women leaving prison. (The third Foundation-supported project was under the Opening Doors program, a collaborative effort with the Henry J. Kaiser Family Foundation that funded projects attempting to lower social and cultural barriers to health care services.)

This chapter, written by Digby Diehl, a best-selling author who has contributed chapters on a wide range of topics to previous volumes of The Robert Wood Johnson Foundation *Anthology*, highlights the passion and charisma of Martha Ryan, the founder and executive director of the Homeless Prenatal Program. Ryan was named a Robert Wood Johnson Community Health Leader in 2003. Diehl makes the point that viability in the nonprofit world requires both the hard work and creativity of individuals such as Ryan and financial support from funders.

He ends the chapter by raising the question of whether programs like the Homeless Prenatal Program can be replicated widely or whether they depend on unique local circumstances and charismatic leaders. It is an important question with which The Robert Wood Johnson Foundation and other foundations continue to grapple.

---

1. See Wielawski, I. M. "The Local Initiative Funding Partners Program." In *To Improve Health and Health Care 2000: The Robert Wood Johnson Foundation Anthology.* San Francisco: Jossey-Bass, 2000.

—ɯ— On any given night, between seven hundred thousand and eight hundred thousand people are homeless in the United States.[1] On an annual basis, between 2.5 million and 3.5 million people in America are estimated to be homeless. Approximately half of the people in these estimates are families with children.[2] Families are the fastest-growing segment of the homeless population.[3] Furthermore, many homeless families are headed by a female facing multiple challenges, including substance abuse, physical and mental disabilities, histories of abuse and violence.[4]

"Family homelessness is a growing national tragedy," says Ellen Bassuk, founder and president of the National Center on Family Homelessness and associate professor of psychiatry at Harvard Medical School. "It is a new social problem, and has grown exponentially in the last twenty years. It is most serious in our urban areas. For example, it is estimated that in New York City, 75 percent of the homeless population are families." Offering an analysis of why there has been such a rapid growth in homeless families, Bassuk explains, "There has been a dramatic increase in female-headed families, and these tend to be the poorest and most vulnerable to becoming homeless."

A 1997 study of 436 homeless and low-income families with female heads found that the mothers in the study had an average age of twenty-seven and had two children. They were extremely impoverished in comparison with the national income norms (about half survived on less than $7,000 a year) and were socially isolated. "A staggering 92 percent of the homeless and 82 percent of the housed [low-income] mothers experienced severe physical and/or sexual assaults at some point in their lives," according to the study. "More than 40 percent in both groups were sexually molested as children. By the age of twelve, 60 percent had been severely physically or sexually abused."[5]

To confront this problem at the local level, an outreach and support network for homeless families, the Homeless Prenatal Program, was founded in San Francisco in 1989. Since its beginning, with one nurse practitioner named Martha Ryan personally providing prenatal care for homeless women in one shelter, the program has expanded into a $1.7

million organization of thirty employees that offers a support network of services and guidance to 1,800 homeless families throughout the city.

Ryan says that there is a long tradition of volunteerism in her family. "We lived in Japan for much of my youth, and my mother volunteered in the hospitals to care for American soldiers injured in the Vietnam War," she said. "I remember learning to knit clothing in Catholic school so that we would have something to give to the poor. After I graduated from the University of San Francisco, I had no idea what I would do with my life, but I loved to travel, so I decided to apply for the Peace Corps. When they told me I was being sent to Ethiopia, I don't think I could even find it on a map. After two years of teaching English in beautiful villages to those beautiful people, my life was changed forever. I came back to study nursing because I wanted to give something more substantial to Africa than English lessons. While I was back here working on my nursing degree, I discovered a whole population of homeless pregnant women who needed my help right here in San Francisco."

Today, although the program no longer offers direct medical care, it has become a comprehensive system of supports for poor families. In addition to family counseling and referral to prenatal care, it works with clients to provide food, housing, parenting education, substance abuse assistance, and advocacy within the courts and Child Protective Services. There are no requirements and no charges for these services. They are provided to any woman who asks for or is willing to accept help from the program. The program is unusual in that it acts as a link that has been missing in the homeless support network: it is a way to penetrate the barriers between women on the streets—who are often confused, addicted, and frightened—and the programs designed to assist them, which are often cold, bureaucratic, and difficult to access. The long-term aim of the Homeless Prenatal Program is to break cycles of poverty, incarceration, and homelessness, and to help each family to build a healthy and stable life.

## —ᨆ— The Genesis of the Homeless Prenatal Program

The Homeless Prenatal Program originated in the Hamilton Family Center in the Haight-Ashbury district, which in 1988 was San Francisco's only city-funded family shelter for the homeless. "It was just a bunch of good-hearted people at the Hamilton Church who fixed up the basement so that anyone who was homeless could find a mattress," recalls Marian Peña, who volunteered at the shelter with Martha Ryan in the late 1980s. "Hamilton was really bare bones. You showed up, you got a bed when you needed it. No questions asked. Martha and I were both working at the Southeast Health Center, going to school, and volunteering at the shelter. Martha saw the surprising number of pregnant women coming to the shelter and decided to do something about it on the spot." With Peña and another colleague, Mary Kate Connor, Ryan set up a prenatal clinic in a one-hundred-square-foot closet in the Hamilton Family Center. The cramped quarters and suspicious, resistant clients made it difficult to provide continuing prenatal care under the auspices of a city program called "Health Care for the Homeless." Because the clinic could see this highly transient population only on a part-time basis, it was hard for the volunteers to maintain contact with a woman throughout her pregnancy.

"Initially, there were three pregnant women that I began to treat at the shelter," Ryan says. "All we had was space for an examination table and a door to close for privacy. I had a Doppler for ultrasound and a stethoscope and could perform a basic prenatal exam. But there wasn't even a sink. More pregnant women came for services, and many of these women were not even staying at the shelter. Some of these women had previously resided at the shelter, but could no longer do so because the shelter limited stays to thirty days. Even when staying elsewhere, these women still came back to the shelter to receive prenatal care. This was also true of women who had left the shelter amid some controversy, which was not uncommon."

"The number of homeless pregnant women came as such a surprise," Ryan remembers. "In fact, the first time I was told that there were homeless pregnant women, I said, 'How can that be?' Of course, it didn't take long to figure out that if a woman was homeless, she would be poor. If she was poor, she wouldn't have health care, but she still would be having sex and so she would get pregnant. After that first year when we saw seventy-two pregnant women, it was clear that there were a lot more homeless pregnant women out there than I could deal with in my little closet clinic. We knew that we had to move to a larger, more neutral space."

During that first year, Ryan also had an insight that became one of the cornerstones of the Homeless Prenatal Program. She saw that pregnancy could be a window of opportunity in a woman's life—a turning point focused on the new responsibilities of motherhood. "Many of these women had poor self-esteem and self-destructive tendencies," Ryan recalls, "but I never met one who did not want to have a healthy baby." She decided that the Homeless Prenatal Program could capitalize on this opportunity—could help women break drug habits, find jobs, end abusive relationships, and become good mothers.

While working at San Francisco General Hospital and volunteering at the Hamilton Center, Ryan was simultaneously studying for her master's degree in public health at the University of California, Berkeley. For a class in grant writing, she wrote a practice grant proposal on homeless prenatal care and sent it off to the only foundation she had ever heard of, the San Francisco Foundation. It landed on the desk of a program officer, Ruth Brousseau. "I was stunned when I got Martha's proposal," Brousseau says. "No one else had ever addressed the problem so directly. I set up a meeting with Martha and helped her to revise her grant proposal. She had asked for $150,000 a year for each of three years, but I knew that the San Francisco Foundation couldn't fund her for that much; so we pared her initial proposal down to $52,000 a year for three years. I advised her to start small, prove that the program could work, and then expand." The board approved the grant; by 1990 the clinic was serving 150 homeless pregnant women, and its resources were overtaxed. Ryan and her associates were frustrated by women being asked to leave the shelter before delivery and finding that it was increasingly difficult to maintain contact with women living transient lives.

## ~w~ The Homeless Prenatal Program Moves to a New Level

In the spring of 1992 the Homeless Prenatal Program registered with the Internal Revenue Service to become a 501(c)(3) nonprofit organization and was preparing to move into a larger location. The program had reached a level where the San Francisco Foundation's Brousseau encouraged it to apply for a Robert Wood Johnson Foundation grant. With the help of

Brousseau and the program's new administrative director, Julia Velson, the San Francisco Foundation nominated the program for a grant from The Robert Wood Johnson Foundation's Local Initiative Funding Partners program. The Robert Wood Johnson Foundation was joined by three others—the James Irvine Foundation, the California Tamarack Foundation, and the Koret Foundation—to provide matching grant dollars. These local foundation partners are significant because the Local Initiative program is a national matching grant program that seeks to establish partnerships with foundations in the community in order to provide a stable local funding base.

"The Local Initiative Funding Partners program is very much about its name," says Pauline Seitz, the program's director. "These are local grants; they are for community-based organizations ready to take initiative by adopting a proactive approach to a local problem; and it is very much about the funding partnerships. The Homeless Prenatal Program is a good example. A strong local leader was recognized by four foundations in San Francisco who brought the nomination forward with matching dollars, which makes The Robert Wood Johnson Foundation only one of many funders. Our role was to be part of the root money for this program. We went there when the seed of an idea had already been planted. We were able to provide it with half of a stable funding base for four years. When we left, the root system was in place, and the program has continued to blossom."

Seitz recalls, "I was impressed by this grant proposal from the beginning. They not only met the programmatic criteria, but there was also a certain spark to their plans that I recognized as a strong local initiative. Most powerfully, what I heard in that application was the authentic voice of the community being served."

The proposal requested a $325,000 matching grant over three years in order to pursue a list of specifically defined objectives, among which were the following:

- To extend outreach and services citywide, focusing on street outreach, additional shelters, and preventive outreach in low-income neighborhoods

- To develop a formal community health worker training program and increase the number of community health workers
- To establish postpartum follow-up
- To strengthen and formalize a multidisciplinary provider and referral network
- To relocate to centrally situated offices, thus increasing access to its services
- To complete its transformation to an independent, nonprofit, tax-exempt entity and initiate long-term development and planning
- To develop and implement a rigorous program evaluation

At the time of the application, the staff of the Homeless Prenatal Program consisted of Ryan, an administrator, three social workers, and three community health workers—almost all part-time. As a supplement to the San Francisco Foundation grant, the program had received the Intensive Care for Our Neighbor, or ICON, Award from the St. Joseph Health System in Orange, California. In addition to a significant financial boost, this award gave special recognition to the program's efforts, since it was given to only three organizations nationally that serve marginalized and underserved communities. As explained in the 1992 proposal, the Homeless Prenatal Program was limited in its initial efforts: "Over the past two years, the Homeless Prenatal Program has provided basic prenatal assessment, group and individual counseling, referral for full-scale prenatal care, including care for high risk women, substance abuse counseling and a host of other necessary services."

Despite an admitted failure of data gathering (notes were kept on four-by-six file cards in a box), the two-year pilot period of prenatal services to homeless women had generated encouraging results. Of the twenty women who gave birth in the first ten months of 1990, 90 percent delivered babies of normal birth weight, and 50 percent of those mothers who had previously been substance abusers delivered drug-free babies. In the first ten months of 1991, thirty-three mothers gave birth in the pilot project, with 91 percent of babies having normal birth weight and 70 percent of babies drug free.

Once the Robert Wood Johnson Local Initiative Funding Partners program's matching grant for $325,000 was approved, the Homeless Prenatal Program moved quickly to accommodate a larger staff, to put better financial controls in place, and to reconsider the organizational structure. "During our initial site visit, we urge each of our projects to develop a strategic business plan, and we provide technical assistance," Pauline Seitz notes. "Almost every small nonprofit needs to do work in this area. I know that business planning was particularly helpful to Martha in thinking through the growth of the organization."

Martha Ryan agrees. "In 1992 there were three of us sort of running the Homeless Prenatal Program as a triumvirate," she recalls. "The three were Marian Peña, an ex-nun and very committed social worker, Julia Velson, who was our first administrator, and myself, as our nurse practitioner. For about a year we shared decisions, but the board felt that there should be a central person to be in charge. It was really my vision, so I became the administrator. I was not entirely comfortable in that role because I don't like conflict and I am troubled if I hurt people's feelings by disagreeing, but I'm getting better at it."

## The Community Health Worker Concept on the Streets of San Francisco

When I finished my drug treatment program, I had already been coming to Homeless Prenatal support groups for about a year. I felt pretty good about myself and began to search for a job. I had wanted to be a nurse, but with a jail record and no permanent address, I was ready to do anything. I just walked the streets knocking on doors and looking for work. I went to Wendy's. I went to Ross. I tried at big companies and little stores. One afternoon at the end of another day walking around the city filling out applications, I was on Market Street and thought I might as well go in to see my counselor at Homeless Prenatal. By the time I saw her, I was in tears. I told her that I had been up and down the streets and was feeling exhausted and discouraged. "Why don't you sign up for our community health worker training?" she suggested. I didn't even know what it was. But when I learned that I would have the chance to give back to other people the opportunities that Homeless Prenatal gave me, I couldn't believe it. Now I love what I do because I see people making their lives better every day.

*Carla Roberts, director of the Substance Abuse*
*Services Project and a former client*

During Ryan's ten years as a nurse, she had made intermittent trips to do relief work in Africa, eventually returning to the United States with the intent of becoming a nurse practitioner so that she could work in maternal and child health programs in the developing world. Even as she formulated her ideas for prenatal care of homeless women in San Francisco, her thoughts had turned to Africa. "When I had been in Sudan and Somalia, we trained local women to be the health care providers of the community because they were able to reach the other women and the families we needed to treat," she says. "They really made the difference in preventing epidemics and getting health care to the entire village because they were trusted. I saw the same opportunity in San Francisco to educate formerly homeless women to be community health workers. They had the same knowledge of the homeless 'villages' and could develop trusting relationships far more effectively than health care professionals just walking into the situation. As a bonus, they got some work experience and some self-esteem and the feeling of giving back to their communities. So I decided to model my program after the work I had done in Africa."

On Market Street the Homeless Prenatal Program became more proactive. With three community health workers recruited from the ranks of former clients, Ryan went to the shelters, to the hospitals, to the single-room occupancy hotels, to the bus stations, and to the streets of San Francisco. She found homeless pregnant women who would not go to anyone "official" for help because they were afraid that the Child Protective Services would take their children away. She found immigrant women with citizenship problems that prevented them from seeking assistance. She found women with substance abuse, psychological, and domestic violence issues. Most important, she found women who were ignorant about pregnancy and child care and ignorant of the services and agencies available to help them. In her own assuring, nonjudgmental way, she and her community health workers allayed the fears of these women, found them food and housing, and developed an ongoing relationship of trust and counseling. Those relationships allowed the clients to break away from their self-destructive habits and to raise healthy families.

"I asked my staff—women who were formerly homeless—to make presentations at the San Francisco hospitals and clinics," Ryan says. "They talked about what it was like to come into the clinic and have somebody snub them or have someone look at them and start second-guessing who they were without trying to know them. It worked well to get clients referred to us and gave a little sensitivity training to the hospital staffs." Quickly, the program had dozens of clients, and by 1994 it had 142 women as clients, 110 of whom were pregnant. That year, the program also hired Ramona Woodruff, who had been one of the Homeless Prenatal Program's first clients and had gone on to work for the program, to be the full-time supervisor and trainer of the community health workers.

As the Homeless Prenatal Program developed, it began to work more closely with other providers of services for homeless women and began to advise women on possibilities for improving their lives. "The Homeless Prenatal Program is one of the best organizations we work with," says Mildred Crear, director of maternal and child health for the City and County of San Francisco. "They are able to locate pregnant women and gain their trust in ways that government agencies have not been able to do. By bringing their clients to the appropriate agencies for food, housing, and health services, the Homeless Prenatal Program allows us to help homeless and needy people early with preventive medicine and education so that they do not develop more serious and more expensive medical problems later. They have also helped us to improve our services. We administer a federal supplemental food voucher program called 'Women, Infants, and Children,' or WIC, and one of the first things Martha pointed out to us was that these women had little or no access to food storage. Significant portions of large containers of milk and bread and cheese would go to waste, because pigeons would eat food left on window sills for refrigeration, or milk would go bad inside, or rats would find food before it could be consumed. We were able to work with the state to have the WIC packets resized so that families could have fresh food more frequently."

"From that experience," Crear explains, "we looked around at the state level and realized that other counties in California didn't have any programs like Homeless Prenatal Program. In 1995, we implemented a Homeless Prenatal Conference, cosponsored by five counties who network and share resources for homeless women and families. The conference has met successfully for the past seven years. Also, I have now been able to provide a public health nurse to be housed at the San Francisco Department of Human Services, so that every pregnant woman who comes in to sign up for benefits is interviewed and referred to Homeless Prenatal Program, as well as to our services."

By the spring of 1994, the Homeless Prenatal Program had grown to a staff of twelve, with five community health workers who worked with clients on a daily basis. All of the community health workers were being trained by a full-time health educator, with instruction in the prevention of sexually transmitted diseases, medical risks during pregnancy, family planning, and mental health techniques. They also learned peer counseling, computer skills, résumé writing, interviewing techniques, and other employment preparation skills.

## —w— The Substance Abuse Services Project

According to the National Clearinghouse for Alcohol and Drug Information, "Data from one study of 36 hospitals, mainly in urban areas, were extrapolated to arrive at an estimate of 375,000 infants exposed *in utero* to illegal drugs each year, or 11 percent of all births."[6] Despite this real problem, there were no treatment programs available to women.

Ramona Woodruff, the supervisor and coordinator of community health workers at the Homeless Prenatal Program, had played an important role in advocating for programs to assist drug-addicted pregnant women while she was still one of the program's early clients. "We had not really looked into the relationship between the use of crack cocaine and high-risk pregnancy until the late 1980s," says Catherine Dodd, a nurse who was the director of women's services at San Francisco General Hospital in 1988, when she met Martha Ryan. (She is now an assistant to Representative Nancy Pelosi.) "We knew about fetal alcohol syndrome, but this was new. I suggested that a group of perinatal advocates go to Sacramento to explain the problem to our elected officials."

"In 1989," Dodd recalls, "Martha, Ellie Journey from the March of Dimes, Ramona Woodruff, and I met with Jackie Speier, who was then an assemblywoman and is now a state senator. Ramona spoke emotionally about her struggle with crack cocaine addiction. She had been sober for ninety days at that point, and the Homeless Prenatal Program had given her hope and changed her life. Speier was deeply moved and immediately picked up the telephone and spoke with the governor. She said, 'We must do something about prenatal substance abuse. It is inexcusable that all of the substance abuse programs are targeted at men and all of the federal funding is targeted at men.'"

Speier wrote and sponsored a bill, Alcohol and Drug Affected Mothers and Infants, which was signed into law by Governor George Deukmejian on September 30, 1990. The law created the Office of Perinatal Substance Abuse within the state Department of Alcohol and Drug Programs and an interagency task force to address the needs of substance-abusing pregnant women.

With state drug treatment programs in place, one of the first extensions of its work with homeless women that the Homeless Prenatal Program was able to develop was the Substance Abuse Services Project. A successfully recovering client, Carla Roberts, was hired to work as a case manager at the program. She was particularly effective in dealing with women who had substance abuse problems. "I got pregnant at seventeen and managed to graduate, and all of that time I was smoking marijuana and selling crack cocaine," she says. "I felt especially bad because I had both of my parents still together and they had stressed the importance of education to their kids. I was still with the guy who had fathered the baby and was starting to take certified nursing assistant classes. I thought I had it together. Eventually, I ended up staying up late getting high on crack cocaine with my own customers, the people I used to feel sorry for. So from there, my whole life just spiraled downhill." Roberts was arrested a number of times on drug and petty theft charges. Fortunately for her, a judge in San Mateo County decided to mandate her to do a year in a drug treatment program instead of six months in jail. The program was called Mothers and Infants Aligning, or MIA, and during the eighteen months at MIA House, Roberts was sent to the Homeless Prenatal Program for counseling. As she continued in the program, she was selected for training as a community health worker and came to work at the program.

"Carla actually went on to become an AmeriCorps volunteer with the Homeless Prenatal Program after she finished her training and became a full-time community health worker. As an AmeriCorps volunteer, she developed a program to help women who were trying to get into drug recovery programs. It was her brainchild, and when her two-year commitment came to a close, she continued on with the Homeless Prenatal Program, overseeing the program as a full-time case manager," Ryan recalls.

Roberts told Ryan that addicts had an especially difficult time obtaining help from government agencies because the system seemed to be set up to discourage them more than to assist them. Roberts pointed out that these women were required to bring government-issued photo ID, find their birth certificates, provide cash or Medi-Cal papers, stand in long lines all day, only to be told that they were in the wrong line, and check in every day on the telephone. "Before I agreed to start our own substance abuse services project, I actually went down to stand on the line myself at the San Francisco Department of Human Services," Ryan recalls. "The people were very slow and impersonal. Now, I'm a white woman and not a drug user, but that made no difference. They didn't care. I have been there many times since trying to help clients to obtain benefits, and they have not become any less impersonal. Virtually the only way an addicted woman, already living a chaotic life, could jump through the hoops required to enter a government drug recovery program would be if someone helped her."

This is what the Homeless Prenatal Program's Substance Abuse Services Project does. It is now composed of four women, including Roberts, who help addicted women to understand the diversity of drug treatment programs that are available and to find one that they are willing to enter. In addition to the preparatory paperwork and communications obligations, the staff of the Substance Abuse Services Project realized that most of these drug treatment programs require financial contributions to the cost of treatment. They have been working to provide clients—who are usually jobless as well as homeless—with employment opportunities. Private meetings with case management workers are supplemented by weekly support group meetings for women to meet others who are dealing with similar problems.

## —∿— The Perinatal Services Project

"One aspect of the Homeless Prenatal Program's development has been the growing awareness that homeless motherhood is not a single, simple issue. It is a complicated collection of problems," says Nancy Frappier, coordinator of the program's Perinatal Services Project. "Martha quickly understood that in addition to prenatal care, homeless pregnant women need help to continue to care for the baby after birth. In 1995 she conceived of what she called the 'Aftercare Project,' obtained a three-year grant under the Opening Doors Project, and hired me."

Opening Doors: Reducing Sociocultural Barriers to Health Care was a joint program, established in 1992, of The Robert Wood Johnson Foundation and the Henry J. Kaiser Family Foundation. The foundations allocated $5.5 million to focus on ways to provide health care to people with issues of culture, language, race, or ethnicity. In their call for proposals, the two foundations noted that "even when health care is available and affordable, certain groups face non-financial obstacles to care, resulting in poorer access to care and health outcomes among racial and ethnic minority groups in the United States." The Perinatal Services Project, which primarily connected impoverished or homeless black and Hispanic families to health care and parenting services, fit the Opening Doors requirements. Although funding from the two foundations ended, the Homeless Prenatal Program has continued the Perinatal Services Project with funding from other sources.

"Our focus is working with a pregnant woman in her last trimester of pregnancy and then after the birth of the baby," Frappier notes. "We support these women in having healthy families, and we try to work with them until the child reaches the age of five." The program offers an ongoing series of training sessions for baby care, parenting, and prenatal education. Case management counselors assist new mothers in obtaining cribs, baby food, breast pumps, diapers, and other basics for newborns. In many instances, case managers also act as liaisons or advocates for clients with the Child Protective Services or court systems. In addition to Frappier, there are two staff members and student interns from San Francisco State in the social work program and volunteer nursing students.

One component of the Opening Doors proposal was the establishment of a Policy Advisory Group, a panel that shared information about homeless prenatal care with other groups and tried to provide information for policymakers. "Most direct service organizations don't make policy at all, but part of my background was the political action side, so I was attracted to this immediately," Frappier says. "I felt excited about bringing those things together"—service and policy change. The Policy Advisory Group evolved into the Advocacy/Policy Program, which continues to inform legislators and health care policymakers on homeless family issues and also works on individual cases. One of the most important victories for the policy group was an allocation of $360,000 by the San Francisco Board of Supervisors to replace housing funds for homeless families that the federal government had eliminated.

## —w— Reshaping the Board of Directors

As the Homeless Prenatal Program grew larger and reached out further into the homeless community with its programs, members of its board, Local Initiative's Pauline Seitz, and other supporters were urging Martha Ryan to step up to another level of professionalism in management, fundraising, and business organization. As a result, in the mid-1990s, the program added new board members from the private sector. One of the new members was Gil Fleitas, a real estate executive. "My business partner, Steven Mavromihalis, who was president of the Homeless Prenatal Program's board, asked me to join the board shortly after I moved from New York to San Francisco," Fleitas recalls. "After attending board meetings for about a year, I began to question what I was doing. I was very successful in my professional career, but I wasn't doing anything to make the world a better place. I wasn't feeling fulfilled. In the summer of 1998, I made the decision to devote myself to volunteer work, primarily with Homeless Prenatal Program. Shortly thereafter, Steven asked me if I would consider taking over as president of the board."

Fleitas, a soft-spoken man with a genial manner, set to work bringing the tools of private sector management into the Homeless Prenatal Program—"without destroying the culture." Gently strengthening concepts such as financial discipline, strategic planning, succession planning, and measurement of results made the Homeless Prenatal Program a stronger organization. "There were a couple of board meetings in which some people were horrified that I would even mention such issues," Fleitas recalls. "I assured them that if we didn't ask the hard questions of ourselves, the people who were funding us would ask them." Both Fleitas and Ryan admit that there was a clash between the older board members with strong feelings about protecting the character of the Homeless Prenatal Program and the new, business-oriented members. Thanks to Fleitas's patience and willingness to compromise, the board members navigated through some contentious meetings to find agreement. In 2000, the fourteen-member board won the Lighthouse Award for excellence in nonprofit management from the Management Center in San Francisco.

## The Jail Outreach Project

I was a young mother at sixteen, and I got married at seventeen to an older man. I stayed with him for five years, but it was a domestic violence situation and I just walked out one day with my two children and not a dollar in my pocket. A friend gave us a place to sleep, but I couldn't find work. The Hispanic culture can be very harsh toward women. My family turned their backs on me. My father said I had it coming. Now my husband and his family have my children because I didn't know where to turn. I didn't know where to go. I was lost. I was depressed. I turned to drugs and prostitution. I ended up in jail.

That's why I have so much passion for this job. I thank God for putting me here. I'm trying to give these women the help I never got. Sometimes it is hard because I miss my children so much. It is so wonderful to see mothers reunited with their children. One day I want to do that. One day I want to have my children back.

*Maria Enriquez (a pseudonym), community health worker with the Jail Outreach Project*

Perhaps the most daring step in a series of innovative programs at the Homeless Prenatal Program is the Jail Outreach Project. The problem being addressed is a daunting one. Women are the fastest-growing segment of the incarcerated population.[7] The number of women in California prisons has tripled over the past decade. The national female prisoner population has more than doubled since 1990. Women are the least violent component of the inmate population. More than 85 percent of women in jail are charged with nonviolent offenses. Women incarcerated for domestic violence offenses are frequently charged with fighting back against an abusive mate.

Carla Roberts, the initiator and administrator of the Substance Abuse Services Project, had many discussions with Martha Ryan about the damaging effects on homeless women of jail sentences for minor offenses, and she spoke from experience. After Roberts pointed out that the moment of release from jail was a window of opportunity for a woman, much like pregnancy, Ryan sought another grant from The Robert Wood Johnson Foundation's Local Initiative Funding Partners program—this one to help 1,050 incarcerated women who are making the transition from jail back to society. The Knossos Foundation nominated the Homeless Prenatal

Program for a Local Initiative program award, and, in 2000, the program received a three-year $314,000 matching grant. This time The Robert Wood Johnson Foundation partnered with the Knossos Foundation, the San Francisco Foundation, the VanLobenSels/RembeRock Foundation, the Zellerbach Foundation, and the Tesuque Foundation to provide matching grant dollars.

According to Pauline Seitz, "The Homeless Prenatal Program is unusual in having been awarded two different grants. Out of the two hundred programs that have been funded by the Local Initiative program between 1988 and 2002, only two have been funded twice. In each case, they returned for funding of a project that was completely different from the initial application."

The proposal's executive summary succinctly relates the problem addressed by the new project:

> Every year approximately 750 women pass through the portals of the [San Francisco] County Jail. Of these women, 88 percent (660) are homeless and approximately 6 percent are pregnant. According to the Discharge Planning Unit, 90 percent (675) are in jail as the result of behavior that stems from substance abuse. Most are mothers. At the present time, there is virtually no safety net for women exiting jail. Furthermore, because of overcrowded conditions, women are released at all hours of the night. With no place to go, the incidence of recidivism is high.

The caseworkers hired for the Jail Outreach Project are all formerly incarcerated women in recovery, and they are strongly motivated to provide the support that in many cases they never got. There are three primary aspects to their work: first, persuading women in jail that there is an alternative to their previous lives; second, providing transportation by taxi on the night of release and prepaying one night's lodging at a single-room-occupancy hotel two and a half blocks from the Homeless Prenatal Program's office with a twenty-four-hour front desk so the released prisoners have somewhere to go; and third, following through with support once a released woman comes to the Homeless Prenatal Program.

The Jail Outreach Project has performed well in the second and third parts of this effort by finding food, housing, and medications for newly released women, as well as arranging pretreatment counseling, referrals to health services, a weekly support group for addicted women, and a bi-monthly writing workshop. However, convincing newly released women to take advantage of this opportunity to find a new direction in life has proved to be surprisingly difficult.

"We go into the jail twice a week—me, Lupe, Judy, Karen, and Giannina," Roberts says. "When I first started to work in the jails seven years ago, I was seeing women who were between twenty-nine and forty-five. Now, it's eighteen, nineteen, or twenty. These young women are usually very alone and very afraid. We reach out to them and offer a helping hand. If we can make a connection with these women and get them to come to us at the end of their sentence, they have a good chance of staying out and starting a new life. But we see too many who don't take our help and just keep going back to jail. When we talk with the women in jail, we ask what their needs are, what it would take to prevent them from coming back. If they come to us when they get out, we help them to find housing, food, and employment. We go with them to parole meetings or court hearings. It is particularly difficult if a woman has a drug felony because then she is not eligible for public housing, welfare, or financial aid for education. There is a stigma that prevents them from applying for most normal employment. They are getting double the punishment."

Despite its efforts to break the chain of recidivism, the Jail Outreach Project has encountered more resistance to its outreach than it anticipated, and both Ryan and Roberts admit that they have not met their self-imposed goals. "The relationships with boyfriends or drug-oriented social groups that often may have landed these women in jail in the first place are strong ties," Ryan says. "Stronger than we realized. We were too optimistic in our projections of how many women would accept our offers of help. We've developed a good working relationship with the Discharge Planning Unit of the county jail, and we have had success with women who come to us. But too many of these women are into a cycle of hopelessness that we have to figure out how to break."

## —ᙡ— The Future

In fifteen years of development, the Homeless Prenatal Program has grown from that closet in the Hamilton Family Center to an effective outreach

I came here about a year ago because I was homeless and I needed shelter. I was nervous about coming. I'm still nervous. Being on the streets makes you suspicious of everybody. I wasn't pregnant when I came in, but I just gave birth to my son eight days ago; and I was so grateful for all of the support I had from everyone here. I'm taking parenting classes, and I feel like I am going to be a good mother to my son. Before, I just was a hardheaded kid and hung out with the wrong people. I was selling drugs and doing drugs and got arrested for shoplifting. What I was doing then looks pathetic to me now. Lupe has been more than just a counselor to me; she's my best friend. She came after me when I got out of jail and convinced me to come into the Homeless Prenatal Program and helped me find a place to stay and something to eat. She's gone to court with me every time. If she wasn't at my side, I doubt if I would go. If I am in pain, she's there. I know that without her help I would be out on the streets or in jail again. I know that I wouldn't have my baby. Sometimes, I just feel low or lonely, and I come by to see Lupe, and it gives me a lift. Most people can't imagine how terrible it was to be completely alone and to have someone like her to hold out her hand to me.

*Betty Johnson (pseudonym), a Jail Outreach client*

program for homeless women in the San Francisco area. Despite her accomplishments, Ryan has bigger plans yet. "One of my goals is to create a community center where families can come into one place and have all of their needs met," she says. "I want it to be a real public and private one-stop partnership so that representatives from the state and city agencies for the poor can meet their clients in one building. We will provide family counseling, housing assistance, substance abuse services, perinatal classes—all of the work we are already doing. I'd like to see legal services and immigration help and computer training and child care and exercise classes. Most of all, I would like to establish a community health clinic in the building where families can get simple health care services and prenatal examinations.

It would be a place where children could get vaccinations and adults could have mental health services. I'd like to run that clinic." She stops for a few moments and then turns back to reality. "We've already got a design and a property. Now, all we need is $6 million to build it."

Gil Fleitas added another, perhaps more important, goal. "When I first joined the board of the Homeless Prenatal Program and saw what they were doing and saw how effective it was and saw the difference that it was making in people's lives, the first thought that popped into my head was, 'What a shame that it is only here. Why can't this be elsewhere?'" Although many urban areas have family shelters, homeless prenatal programs, family counseling centers, low-cost housing programs, drug treatment centers, and other services, nowhere outside of San Francisco's Homeless Prenatal Program is there a comprehensive service and support system for women and families in crisis. Ellen Bassuk, of the National Center on Family Homelessness, observes, "I am not aware of another program with the comprehensive scope of services that the Homeless Prenatal Program provides. I wish there were many of them."

According to Pauline Seitz, the issue of re-creating some of the innovative programs from the Local Initiative program's grants has grown in importance for her, too. "The Local Initiative grants come to us because they are strong models in their communities. Many of them are led by passionate, charismatic leaders like Martha Ryan, who seem to be one of a kind in their energy, dedication, and vision. But we need to learn how to disseminate what they do."

When Fleitas became president of the Homeless Prenatal Program board, he strongly recommended to Ryan that she have a succession plan and that she needed to codify the intervention techniques of her community health workers. "I said to her, 'You've created this wonderful organization with concepts and operating principles and a culture that works. Why not figure out how to make it work in other cities? Why not figure out how to put the Homeless Prenatal Program in a box?'" he recalls with a laugh. "We may never find another Martha Ryan, but we can teach others how to do what you have done."

"I'll never forget the first time Gil talked to me about this issue," Ryan says. "I was taken aback. My first thought was that I must have been doing an inadequate job. But when I calmed down, I realized that he was absolutely correct—a good leader is only as good as the organization is when he or she is gone. Not only should this organization continue and thrive if anything ever happened to me, I would love to share what we have learned. I would love to see the Homeless Prenatal Program replicated all over the world. We have been working on succession planning and writing down the steps we go through with our clients and the lessons learned. We still have a long way to go. And I have added another goal to my dreams for the future of Homeless Prenatal Program. Someday I want to see one of our former clients, a woman from the streets or the jail, become president of this organization. That's really when we will have achieved a big victory for homeless families."

## Notes

1. *Who Is Homeless?* Fact Sheet, no. 3. National Coalition for the Homeless, Sept. 2002. (http://www.nationalhomeless.org/education/families.html).
2. Burt, M. R., and Aaron, L. Y. *America's Homeless II: Populations and Services.* The Urban Institute, Feb. 1, 2000. (http://www.urban.org/uploadedPDF/900344_AmericasHomelessII.pdf); *Homeless Families with Children.* Fact Sheet, no. 7. National Coalition for the Homeless, June 2001. (http://www.nationalhomeless.org/education/families.html).
3. Ibid.
4. Rog, D. J., and Gutman, M. "The Homeless Families Program: A Summary of Key Findings." In *To Improve Health and Health Care 1997: The Robert Wood Johnson Foundation Anthology.* San Francisco: Jossey-Bass, 1997.
5. "WFRP: The Worcester Family Research Project." The National Center on Family Homelessness, 2003. (http://www.familyhomelessness.org/research_evaluation/research.html).
6. *Pregnant, Substance-Using Women: Treatment Improvement Protocol (TIP), Series 2.* National Clearinghouse for Alcohol and Drug Information, 1993. (http://www.health.org/govpubs/bkd107/2d.aspx); Freier, M. C., Griffith, D. R., and Chasnoff, I. J.

"In Utero Drug Exposure: Developmental Follow-Up and Maternal-Infant Interaction." *Seminars in Pathology,* 1991, *15*(4), 310–316.

7. Irwin, J., Schiraldi, V., and Ziedenberg, J. *America's One Million Nonviolent Prisoners.* Washington, D.C.: Justice Policy Institute, 1999, pp. 6–7. Cited in "Drug War Facts: Women and the Drug War." Apr. 29, 2003. (http://www.drugwarfacts.org/women.htm).

# Pioneering Portfolio

# 10

# The Robert Wood Johnson Foundation's Response to Emergencies

## September 11th, Bioterrorism, and Natural Disasters

*Stephen L. Isaacs*

---

### Editor's Introduction

This chapter by Stephen Isaacs, coeditor of The Robert Wood Johnson Foundation *Anthology,* examines how the Foundation has responded to emergencies that take lives and threaten the public's health. The most traumatic event was the terrorist attacks of September 11, 2001, but natural disasters (such as earthquakes and hurricanes) and bioterrorism (for example, the 2001 anthrax attacks) are situations that also require an emergency response. Isaacs explores all three situations.

For a foundation such as The Robert Wood Johnson Foundation, which is focused on long-range and highly targeted goals, responding to immediate emergencies—particularly of the scale of September 11th—raises profound issues. For example, should the foundation aim simply at helping agencies cope with emergencies, or should it relate its assistance to the Foundation's priorities? Should it take the lead or wait to see what others do and then look for a niche? Should it work alone or jointly with others?

A key issue—one that affects the philanthropic sector as a whole—is the role of foundations in situations where the support of others becomes overwhelming. For example, September 11th brought forth an enormous outpouring of charitable giving by individuals, foundations, corporations, and the U.S. government. Similarly, the anthrax-laced letters mailed shortly after September 11th and the threat of subsequent bioterrorist attacks triggered a huge federal investment in states' emergency preparedness systems. Isaacs explores how the Foundation struggled to carve out a role for itself in these circumstances and analyzes where foundations can fit in when the resources of others have the potential of preempting the field.

Although this chapter emphasizes the institutional response of The Robert Wood Johnson Foundation to September 11th and other emergencies, the personal response of staff members should not be forgotten. In the immediate aftermath of September 11th, senior program officer Susan Hassmiller, a nurse and member of the board of the American Red Cross, volunteered her time to help organize the relief effort and did not return to work for another two weeks. Administrative assistant Sheri DeMarchi organized donations of food, clothing, and other needed items. Other staff members gave money, blood, and time. The staff wanted to help in whatever way it could, and it did so well beyond the institutional response that Isaacs chronicles in the following pages.

J.R.K.

—ɯ— Septemberber 11, 2001. The mood at The Robert Wood Johnson Foundation's headquarters in Princeton, New Jersey, that morning was somber, bewildered, shocked, disbelieving. By 9:00 A.M., many of the Foundation's staff members were gathering in small groups around television sets in three of the Foundation's conference rooms. They watched as the second plane hit the North Tower, both of the Twin Towers imploded, a third plane crashed into the Pentagon, and a fourth crashed in a field outside of Pittsburgh. They talked in whispered tones, wondering how many planes were still in the air, how many had been hijacked, and, most important, whether any friends, colleagues, or loved ones had lost their lives. People called their wives, husbands, parents, children, and friends. Some went home to be with them. Many stayed at the office, alternately watching the television, listening to the radio, talking with colleagues, listlessly trying to get some work done, taking consolation in the presence of their coworkers. A call came from the husband of a former staff member who was working in one of the towers; she was safe. The four staff members who were traveling on September 11 called in to say that they, too, were safe. Toward the end of the day, Steven Schroeder, the Foundation's president at the time, went from office to office—talking to each member of the staff, offering words of encouragement, or, sometimes, just a pat on the arm.

The next day, at around noon, Schroeder called together the "management group"—the Foundation's senior leadership consisting of its vice presidents and other officers—to discuss how the Foundation should respond to this horrific event. As might be expected after such a catastrophe, the discussion was free-flowing and inconclusive. Schroeder appointed Nancy Kaufman and Paul Jellinek, vice presidents of the Foundation at the time, to head a task force charged with seeking and sifting through ideas, finding out what others were doing and what the gaps were, and coming up with a response appropriate to the scale of the tragedy and the Foundation's expertise.

That afternoon, the entire staff met in the Foundation's amphitheater. It was standing room only as Jellinek and Kaufman summarized the management group discussions about how the Foundation could respond to the tragedy. The staff quickly jumped in with their ideas. Make sure our grantees in the areas are OK. See who needs additional help. Work to avoid a backlash against Americans of Arab descent. Make sure that disadvantaged people affected by the tragedy are taken care of. Remember the Oklahoma City bombing where the mental health needs of people affected by the trauma lasted many years. Schroeder concluded the meeting by observing how proud he was of the quality and the compassion of the staff; how, in this time of great crisis, it had come together as a family; and how, in the rush to do something special for the victims of September 11th, staff members should remember, and take pride in, the work they do every day to improve the well-being of their fellow Americans. He urged all of the Foundation's staff members to pass their thoughts on next steps to colleagues on the task force.

This was not, of course, the first time the Foundation had been called upon to aid victims of a disaster. Over the years, the Foundation has contributed to the relief efforts of organizations aiding victims of natural disasters such as earthquakes, hurricanes, floods, and tornadoes. Nor was it the last. The anthrax attacks that followed shortly after September 11 demonstrated the weakness of the nation's public health system to respond to bioterrorism. How to respond to disasters, whether natural or human-made, has raised questions for The Robert Wood Johnson Foundation and, indeed, for all philanthropy—questions such as how to balance a compassionate response to relieve suffering and the need to stick with long-term strategies; whether to play a leadership position or wait to fill in gaps left by others; and what role is left for a foundation after the federal government, the voluntary sector, or individuals have invested huge amounts of money toward addressing a problem. Dealing with questions such as these becomes more important at a time in our nation's history when the threat of terrorism raises the possibility of more, and more horrific, emergencies that may demand the attention of foundations.

## —⁓— The Robert Wood Johnson Foundation's Response to Earlier Emergencies

Most of the Foundation's work in disaster relief prior to September 11th had been in the form of grants to support the relief efforts of the American Red

Cross. "The Robert Wood Johnson Foundation's response has been that of a good neighbor," said Steven Schroeder. "We haven't gone about giving assistance in an organized, systematic way, but that's the nature of disaster relief." In 1989, the Foundation awarded the American Red Cross $10,000 to provide relief to the victims of Hurricane Hugo, which ravaged South Carolina and other states, and $50,000 to aid victims of the Lomo Prieta earthquake in Northern California. In subsequent years, the Foundation continued supporting the Red Cross following natural disasters: $50,000 in the wake of Hurricane Andrew in 1992; $500,000 following the 1993 flooding in the Midwest; $100,000 after tornadoes and torrential rains in 1997 had left thousands of people homeless in eight states (Arkansas, Kentucky, Indiana, Illinois, Ohio, West Virginia, Tennessee, and Mississippi); $100,000 following ice storms that left hundreds and thousands of homes and businesses in the Northeast without power in 1998; $1 million following Hurricane Georges in 1998; and $1 million following Hurricane Floyd in 1999.

Not all of the Foundation's support to relief efforts went to the Red Cross. Typically, following a natural disaster, a Foundation staff member would call grantees in the area to find out whether they needed additional assistance. On the basis of such phone calls, the Foundation gave $238,000 to ASPIRA, a grantee in Puerto Rico under an antidrug program called "Free to Grow," for five emergency assistance centers after Hurricane Hortense had devastated the island in September 1996. Two years later, when Hurricane Georges laid waste the island, the Foundation awarded a $400,000 emergency grant to ASPIRA.

Similarly, in 1997, the Foundation gave more than $500,000 to the Grand Forks, North Dakota, health department and the North Dakota state health department after torrential rains had caused the Red River to break through the dike, water engulfed the entire city of Grand Forks, and nearly all of its fifty thousand residents had to be evacuated.

Perhaps the closest parallel to the attacks of September 11th was the bombing of the Alfred P. Murrah Federal Building in Oklahoma City in 1995. There the Foundation awarded the University of Oklahoma Health Sciences Center $96,000 to learn more about post-traumatic stress syndrome and how best to address it. The Foundation's grant enabled the university to carry out surveys of rescue workers, their families and direct victims of the bombing, and the general population in order to document long-term treatment needs.

If the Oklahoma City bombing taught the Foundation anything important for September 11th, it was, said Steven Schroeder, that "events like these have a long tail. The families of the victims of that tragedy needed counseling for many years after."

But, on the whole, neither the response to the Oklahoma City bombing nor the response to natural disasters offered much in the way of guidance on how The Robert Wood Johnson Foundation could best respond to a tragedy of the size, scale, and immediacy of September 11th.

## —⁓— The Foundation's Response to September 11th

At the Foundation's management group meeting on September 12, Paul Jellinek made an impassioned plea to put $100 million on the table— half to be awarded immediately, half later. "I didn't know exactly how the money should be spent," he recalled. "I just knew that a tragedy the magnitude of September 11th deserved a response of a similar magnitude." At the other end of the spectrum, Nancy Kaufman, a public health nurse by training who oversaw many of the Foundation's emergency response grants, counseled a more cautious approach. "There will be a lot of players," she observed, "and it's not clear how we'll be needed." Based on her past experience, she noted that "everybody rushes in immediately after a disaster, but it's the aftermath that needs attention. You have to think about the long term—what happens after the federal agencies and everybody else has disappeared."

The management group decided not to jump in with $100 million. It was a huge amount of money for a foundation that had already overspent the year's budget. Besides, it wasn't at all clear what the money would go for or whether it would force the Foundation to reduce spending on its traditional priorities. Rather, the management group agreed to request a $5 million authorization from the board (it was quickly approved) and to explore what The Robert Wood Johnson Foundation could do that others weren't doing in the wake of September 11[th]. The small task force led by Jellinek and Kaufman was entrusted with the job of finding gaps in the response to September 11$^{th}$ where the Foundation could make a genuine contribution.

This meant having some idea of what others were doing—not an easy task in the weeks and month following September 11$^{th}$. Schroeder called Susan Berresford, president of the Ford Foundation, Rebecca Rimel, president of the Pew Charitable Trusts, and other foundation heads to find out what their foundations were up to. Other staff members spent many hours on the phone calling grantees—particularly those in New York City—to find out what they were doing and whether they needed additional help.

In fact, although it was not wholly clear in the fog of the time, there was an awful lot going on. Voluntary organizations such as the American Red Cross, the Salvation Army, and Safe Horizon set up operations centers at Pier 94 to provide immediate emergency relief to those victimized by the attacks on the World Trade Center. The Federal Emergency Management Agency, or FEMA, was heavily involved. In fact, the federal government's $21 billion contribution to New York City's recovery through FEMA and other federal agencies dwarfed those of all other funders combined.[1]

On the afternoon of September 11, Lorie Slutsky, president of the New York Community Trust, called Ralph Dickerson, her counterpart at United Way of New York City, and invited him to come downstairs (the two organizations have offices in the same building) to a staff meeting to talk about what to do. "We were the two largest charities funding services in New York City, with different areas of expertise and different funding bases," she recalled. "That all suggested that there might be real synergies in a partnership." By the close of the day, the two had agreed to establish a joint fund—the September 11th Fund.[2]

Foundations swung into action. Within days of the attacks, the Ford Foundation had pledged $5 million to the September 11th Fund and another $5 million for other relief efforts. On September 13, the Lilly Endowment, based in Indianapolis, pledged $30 million to the relief and recovery effort. Other foundations, including corporate foundations, contributed generously. Many donated money to the relief organizations or to the funds set up after September 11$^{th}$. Others targeted areas that were of particular importance to them. The Andrew W. Mellon Foundation, for example, pledged $50 million to assist New York City cultural and performing arts institutions affected by the attacks; the Rockefeller Foundation directed much of its $5 million pledge to support the families of non-English-speaking workers who had lost their jobs; the Citigroup Foundation pledged $15 million to provide college scholarships to the children of victims of the attacks. All told, noncorporate foundations contributed $213 million, while corporations and corporate foundations contributed $622 million.[3]

The September 11th attacks galvanized a public outpouring of unparalleled scope. Sixty-five percent of American households contributed to one of the victims' relief funds.[4] Total contributions reached $2.5 billion; the American Red Cross's Liberty Disaster Fund received some $998 million;[5] the September 11th Fund, $503 million; and the Twin Towers Fund, $108 million.[6] In addition, as part of the airlines bailout bill passed in December 2001, Congress established the September 11th Victim Compensation Fund, which was expected to provide an average of $1.5 million to each of the families of those who died in the attacks.[7]

Amid the confusion that lasted for months after the attacks—rescue workers combing the rubble for body parts, money pouring into the funds, foundations responding to the tragedy in an uncoordinated fashion, uncertainty about what would come next, anthrax attacks—staff members of The Robert Wood Johnson Foundation called new grantees, old grantees, officials of state health departments, and others they knew in order to find projects that were being overlooked or where the Foundation could make a difference.

### *The Foundation's First Grant: A Survey on the Public's Reaction to September 11th*

The Foundation's first grant in response to September 11th was made two weeks later, on September 27. It was for $79,000 to enable the National Opinion Research Center in Chicago to conduct a survey of the public reaction to the attacks that could be useful to the American Red Cross, FEMA, and the government.

### Establishing an Emergency Medicaid Application System

The second grant, for $750,000, was approved on October 30 and went to the United Hospital Fund in New York City. It came about by serendipity rather than calculation. Michael Rothman, a senior program officer at the Foundation, read an article in the September 28 *New York Times* noting that the collapse of the Twin Towers had cut the computer link between the city's Human Resources Administration offices and the state eligibility processing office so that Medicaid applications could no longer be processed. As a result, thousands of poor people in New York City and nearby counties were left without their usual access to health care. Rothman called Kathryn Haslanger, who handled Medicaid coverage issues at the United Hospital Fund, to see what exactly the problem was and whether The Robert Wood Johnson Foundation could be of help.

Haslanger explained that given the breakdown in the system, the federal, state, and city governments had created a temporary Disaster Relief Medicaid program—one that would last only between September 24, 2001, and January 31, 2002—that did away with most of the paperwork. During this four-month period, people could sign up for Medicaid (or a new program for low-income adults—Family Health Plus) with virtually no questions asked or documentation required. However, New York City's Human Resources Administration, charged with operating the program, did not have enough money to carry it out and had requested help from the United Hospital Fund.

If it had not been for the September 11th disaster, the government would never have created a program where people could get Medicaid benefits without any verification of their income or even that they lived in the state. It appeared to be a once-in-a-lifetime natural experiment: Would more people enroll in Medicaid if paperwork and bureaucracy were eliminated? Would they lie to get enrolled? If more people enrolled and fraud was limited, could it be a model for other states?

Haslanger quickly prepared a proposal on behalf of the United Hospital Fund and submitted it to the Foundation. The proposal requested funds for seven components of the Disaster Relief Medicaid program that the city's Human Resources Administration had developed collaboratively with the United Hospital Fund. The Foundation rapidly approved the grant, much of which was directed to spreading the word about the program. The Henry J. Kaiser Family Foundation also contributed to the program's implementation and evaluation.

As it turned out, people flocked to the Disaster Relief Medicaid program. In the four months, 350,000 low-income New Yorkers enrolled—about ten times the volume expected in a typical four-month period.[8] While it is not known how many people falsified their income or place of residence in order to enroll or how many continued once the program ended in February 2002, early statistics indicated that roughly half of those who had enrolled in the emergency plan applied for traditional Medicaid after it ended and that about three-quarters of those applicants qualified for benefits.[9]

### Looking After Mental Health Needs

The September 11th attacks caused psychological trauma that will, no doubt, last for many years. Two grantees under the Foundation's Local Initiative Funding Partners program[10]—one a clinic located in Chinatown, within walking distance of Ground Zero, the other a clinic a little farther uptown serving primarily Latinos—were overwhelmed by the number of requests for counseling. In response to phone calls and follow-up from Foundation staff members, they requested funds so that they could provide additional mental health counseling services. In January 2002, the Foundation awarded $150,000 to each of the clinics. The Foundation later provided $198,000 to the Asian American Federation of New York to assess the mental health services that were being provided and that would be needed by the Chinatown community.

Between January and March 2002, the Foundation awarded three other grants focused on dealing with post-traumatic stress and anxiety after September 11th: to the Families and Work Institute in New York City ($180,000) to enable teachers and child-care workers to help young children cope with their fears resulting from the attacks; to the American Academy of Pediatrics ($100,000) to put together materials on helping children cope with the event into a single on-line "toolkit"; and to the Columbia University School of Social Work ($50,000) to add questions about the impact of September 11th to a survey on individual and family well-being in New York City.

### Informing the Public

Within days of the attacks, Nancy Kaufman called George Hardy, the executive director of the Association of State and Territorial Health Officials, or ASTHO, and asked how the Foundation could be of help. Hardy responded, "We're inundated with requests for information. We can't even return calls to CNN, the *New York Times,* and the *Washington Post.* We need communications help. Fast." The Foundation got in touch with Burness Communications, a consulting firm and Foundation grantee located in Washington, D.C., and asked it to provide whatever help was needed. "In less than an hour," says Hardy, "I got a call from the head of the company, Andy Burness. He sent over two people the very next day. They took over handling calls from the press—made us responsive to the media. They also helped us develop a longer-range strategy. And the amazing thing: the Foundation didn't even ask for a proposal."

### Providing Clothing and Equipment to Workers at Ground Zero

On January 11, 2002, a cold, rainy, and generally miserable winter day, Paul Jellinek read a letter from the Art Science Research Laboratory, Inc., a small nonprofit organization headed by sculptor Rhonda Roland Shearer and her husband, paleontologist Stephen Jay Gould (who died in May 2002). The letter said that police and firefighters at Ground Zero were in desperate need of clothing and equipment, even basics such as boots, goggles, and respirators; that the Art Science Research Lab, which was on Spring Street just seventeen blocks from Ground Zero, was providing them; but that it was running out of money and needed financial support to continue its work. "When I read the letter, I thought, 'This is really different,'" Jellinek recalled. "First of all, it was highly specific. Second, it was cosigned by Stephen Jay Gould, whom I knew, of course, by reputation."

"If it was true, the lack of clothing and equipment was shocking," said Jellinek. "But was it true?" Jellinek asked Sherry DeMarchi, an administrative assistant at the Foundation and head of its Giving Committee, to see if she could find out. DeMarchi made a number of phone calls, among them to a fire chief in Brooklyn who told her, "My guys aren't getting the basics to do the job."

So Jellinek picked up the phone, called Rhonda Shearer, and said he'd like to meet with her as soon as possible. In less than two hours, he was in the Art Science Research Lab warehouse. The place was filled with racks of coats, boots, overalls, respirators, goggles, and the like.

On September 11, Shearer was returning from Europe on an Alitalia flight when the captain announced that there had been an emergency in New York and that all airspace in the United States was closed. "I thought, 'Oh my God. Nuclear war,'" she recalled. "I talked my way into the cockpit. The captain told me that there had not been a nuclear attack but that fires were burning in lower Manhattan. My daughter was there. I was in a controlled panic." Since the U.S. borders were sealed, the plane took a detour and landed in Halifax. Shearer was able to get in touch with her daughter and found out that she was all right.

In fact, her twenty-three-year-old daughter, London Shearer Allen, had been hard at work. Because her mother was a sculptor, Allen knew the importance of using a respirator to filter out dust. And there was a lot of dust at the site of the attacks. She donated the respirators that were at the studio to the rescue workers at Ground Zero and then talked with other sculptors, who willingly donated their respirators. When Shearer arrived home three days later, her warehouse, which by a fortunate coincidence was vacant, was already being used as a supply depot.

"As soon as I got back, I saw that there was a tremendous need," Shearer recalled. "Not just respirators, but hard hats, overalls, spades . . . just about everything." The Rockefeller Foundation came through with a $60,000 emergency grant. Contributions began coming in. Representatives of the fire department, the Port Authority, and the police department put together an equipment list. Shearer and her daughter started stockpiling items, using her studio as a warehouse. She got a pass that allowed her to drive a truck to Ground Zero. Her staff of volunteers dropped in at supply posts manned by the Red Cross, the Salvation Army, and FEMA to find out their immediate needs. She and her staff of volunteers continued making deliveries to the police, firefighters, and Port Authority workers, as well as relatives of the victims searching for remains at Ground Zero and later at Fresh Kills (the site in Staten Island where the debris was brought). When the weather started turning nasty in December, Shearer and her colleagues supplied warm winter clothing. With funds running low, Shearer sent out a letter-proposal to about one hundred charities and foundations—the one that came to Jellinek's attention.

When Jellinek got to Ground Zero with Shearer, the firefighters, police, and Port Authority officers confirmed the problem. The shelves of the supply sheds were either empty or often had the wrong kind of equipment; most important, the firefighters, police, and volunteers were using the equipment supplied by the Art Science Research Lab.

A proposal was brought to The Robert Wood Johnson Foundation's management group the following Monday. On January 23, 2002, the Foundation approved a grant of $700,000 for the Art Science Research Lab.

The grant allowed Shearer and her group to buy several months' worth of clothing, equipment, and supplies. Daniel Nigro, who recently retired as chief of the New York City Fire Department, said, "From the firefighters' perspective, Rhonda and her group were wonderful. We knew we could rely on them. Others came in, helped for a while, and then left; but they stuck with it. They were there for us." Lieutenant Paul Brown of Engine Company 290 in Brooklyn wrote, "In many instances, the Art Science Research Lab quickly and efficiently provided urgently needed equipment and supplies under circumstances where the normal supply channels would have taken days or weeks. They have been able to provide supplies, which are outside the abilities of federal, state, and city agencies to provide. This group has allowed us to continue working without waiting for slow supply deliveries and fighting red tape."

"Slow supply deliveries?" "Red tape?" Given this kind of criticism, it was hardly a surprise that tension developed between Shearer, an outsider doing effective work, albeit in an unorthodox, nonbureaucratic way, and the city's Office of Emergency Management, which was charged with supplying the rescue workers and which, according to the *New York Times,* "when crisis struck, found itself marginalized and overwhelmed."[11] The Office of Emergency Management, whose own command center on the twenty-third floor of 7 World Trade Center had been destroyed on September 11th, viewed Shearer and her group as interlopers, cast doubt on her credibility, and attempted to revoke her credentials.[12] (One observer noted that the Office of Emergency Management might also have resented the Art Science Research Lab's supplying victims' relatives who, in the opinion of some of its officials, shouldn't have been sifting through the rubble in the first place.) For her part, Shearer felt that the Office of Emergency Management simply didn't understand basic supply management. "For God's sake," she said. "They weren't even stockpiling items. They weren't keeping track of shipments. And a lot of the time, they would be satisfied supplying the wrong things." Whatever bad blood might have existed, there are no villains in the story. People were doing their best, forced to "wing it" in an unprecedented, horrific, and evolving situation.

In March 2002, the Art Science Research Lab needed at least $400,000 more to cover costs during April and May, and Shearer came back to The Robert Wood Johnson Foundation. This time the Foundation agreed to provide $100,000 as a challenge grant, with the proviso that the Lab would have to come up with the additional money from other sources. Shortly after, the New York Community Trust agreed to meet the challenge, and awarded $400,000 to the group, which was fortunate, since Shearer had put her property up as collateral to get a loan to buy more supplies for workers at Ground Zero.

### The Foundation's Response to September 11th in Retrospect

Looking back, the easiest thing for the Foundation to do would have been simply to make a donation to the September 11th Fund, much as the Foundation had given money to the American Red Cross following earlier disasters. Originally, the Foundation's task force had planned to do just that—give half of the $5 million to the September 11th Fund. "But we moved cautiously," said former Foundation vice president Paul Jellinek. "We wanted to know how decisions about funding were going to be made and who was going to get funded. By the time we finally received the information that we needed to make a decision, Joshua Gotbaum, the September 11th Fund's chief executive officer at the time, had announced that they had enough money and didn't need any more."

This typifies the posture the Foundation adopted: waiting to see what others were going to do and expecting to fill in the gaps. But because of the outpouring of generosity from the American public, the gaps never appeared, and the Foundation never found a niche. With the exception of those few grants that the Foundation's staff sought out—to the Art Science Research Lab, the United Hospital Fund, and community agencies in the vicinity of Ground Zero, for example—it stayed largely on the sidelines. As a result, it spent only $2 million of the $5 million that had been authorized.

Whether this represents an overly cautious or an appropriately prudent response is a matter of judgment. Many people feel that the Foundation could have done more—that its response to this event that occurred only fifty miles away was not commensurate with the scale of the tragedy. One Foundation program officer expressed it concisely: "The response to September 11th was mainly waiting, waiting, waiting. We were waiting to see where we were needed; we didn't want to just jump in. It was frustrating that we didn't do more. . . . that we couldn't do more."

Others feel that while the Foundation might have played more of a leadership role, such a role wasn't appropriate. Unlike, say, the Ford Foundation, which is located in midtown Manhattan and played a central role, The Robert Wood Johnson Foundation lies more than an hour away. Commenting on the geographical distance, Steven Schroeder said, "There is a real question about how active a leadership role a Princeton-based foundation can and should play in responding to a tragedy like September 11th."

Moreover, there is a question about how much a foundation—any foundation—should deviate from its basic mission in order to respond to an emergency, even one as devastating as that caused by the attacks on the World Trade Center and the Pentagon. The Foundation's decision was, ultimately, not to deviate much from its more strategic approaches to improving Americans' health and health care.

## —⚬— Preparing for Future Emergencies: Bioterrorism and the Public Health System

The events during and following September 2001 posed new questions about how foundations can best support the public health system in the area of disaster preparedness, including readiness for potential bioterrorist attacks. Given its mission to improve health and health care, these questions are particularly relevant for The Robert Wood Johnson Foundation.

### *The Anthrax Attacks of September–October 2001*

Less that a month after the attacks of September 11th, the nation reeled from another kind of terrorism—biological warfare. It began in south Florida. On Monday, October 1, Robert Stevens, a photo editor for the *Sun,* a tabloid in Boca Raton, began to feel ill. By Tuesday he was running a high fever and was incoherent. He began having convulsions. His wife took him to the emergency room of the John F. Kennedy Medical Center in Palm Beach County. Doctors performed a spinal tap. Stevens' spinal fluid was filled with rodlike bacteria that looked initially like anthrax. The diagnosis was tentative since there had been only eighteen cases of inhalation anthrax in the past hundred years, and the last case had been reported a quarter of a century earlier. The state laboratory confirmed the diagnosis of anthrax on October 4. Stevens lapsed into a coma and, on October 5, died of respiratory failure.

Even before Stevens died, a team of investigators from the Centers for Disease Control and Prevention (CDC) was rushed to Boca Raton. Tests of the mailroom at the *Sun* revealed that the mail bin was rich with anthrax spores. The head of the investigative team called the CDC director, Jeffrey Koplan, and reported, "We have evidence for an intentional cause of death of Robert Stevens."[13] The source, apparently, was a letter (never found) sent to the mailroom of the *Sun.* It was followed by a spate of letters containing anthrax spores (analysis of one of the letters revealed that the anthrax was finely milled, making it easy to float and enter the lungs of the victims) sent to, among others, Tom Brokaw at NBC, the

*New York Post,* Senator Tom Daschle, and Senator Patrick Leahy. Many of the letters were mailed in Trenton, New Jersey, and some were sorted in the post office of the township where The Robert Wood Johnson Foundation headquarters is located.

Between September 2001 and January 2002, twenty-two people were infected with anthrax; five of them died. The public health system—the first line of defense against anthrax attacks—was severely strained. Laboratories were pressed to identify thousands of samples of suspicious powders. State and local health departments were inundated with requests for analyses of environmental samples, nasal swabs, and clinical specimens. Thirty-three thousand people were placed on antibiotics. In addition, the anthrax attacks crippled businesses, postal services, and government (the Hart Senate Office Building was closed for more than three months; it cost $23 million to decontaminate it).[14] Moreover, they contributed to the growing sense of vulnerability the nation had felt since September 11th.

The anthrax attacks spotlighted the serious weaknesses in the nation's public health system to cope with a biological terror attack.[15] In a sense, the nation was fortunate that the anthrax was disseminated by means of a few letters. Had it (or, even worse, smallpox) been sprayed from a crop duster over a populated metropolitan area, the death, illness, and disruptions would have been incalculably worse.

In a sense, the anthrax attacks were a shot across the bow. But it was certainly not the first time that biological or chemical agents were used as an instrument of war or terror. Roman armies used infected animal and human corpses to contaminate their enemies' drinking water. During the siege of Kaffa in 1346, the attacking Tartars catapulted plague-infected corpses into the city held by the Genoan army. During the French and Indian War in the mid-1700s, British commander Sir Jeffrey Amherst ordered smallpox-contaminated blankets to be distributed to Delaware Indians. In World War I, mustard gas, chlorine, and phosgene were all used in combat. In World War II, the Japanese military dropped plague-infested fleas over populated areas of China.

More recently, in 1984, members of the Rajneeshee cult contaminated restaurant food in Wasco County, Oregon, with salmonella and poisoned at least 750 people. In 1995, the Aum Shinrikyo religious cult released sarin gas in the Tokyo subway, causing nineteen deaths and thousands of injuries. In 1988, Saddam Hussein's military used chemical weapons (believed to include mustard gas, sarin, and VX) on Kurdish inhabitants of Halabja and Goktapa.[16] Most chilling yet, the former Soviet Union is known to have had programs to develop genetically modified strains of smallpox, plague, and anthrax capable of defeating drugs, antidotes, and vaccines.[17]

### The Public Health System and Bioterrorism

Although the nation's lack of preparation for a biological attack had been recognized as a problem, it was not a top priority before September 11, 2001, but federal, state, and municipal governments were taking some action. For example, between 1998 and 2001, the amount of money in the federal budget earmarked for preparing the nation for, and responding to, chemical, biological, and nuclear attacks rose from $645 million to $1.6 billion—a nearly 150 percent increase.

Notwithstanding this attention, the nation's—and particularly the public health system's—ability to respond to a bioterror attack was weak. As far back as 1988, the Institute of Medicine's Committee for the Study of the Future of Public Health concluded, "The nation has lost sight of its public health goals and has allowed the system of public health to fall into disarray."[18] Two exercises that simulated bioterror attacks—Operation Topoff in May 2000 and Dark Winter in June 2001—showed that leaders were unprepared, crucial information was lacking, vaccines were limited, the health care system was quickly overburdened, and state and federal officials disagreed about who was in charge.[19]

However, it took the events of and after September 11th for the nation to recognize that its public health system is the first line of defense against bioterrorism and that it was still in disarray.[20] Recognizing the importance of addressing the crisis immediately, Congress passed the Public Health Security and Bioterrorism Preparedness and Response Act. Designed to improve the CDC's capacity to deal with bioterrorism, increase the capacity of state and local public health agencies and hospitals, develop a coordinated network of public health labs, conduct research on vaccines, and enhance the government's authority to safeguard the nation's food and water supplies. It was signed into law in June 2002. Six months earlier, in December 2001, Congress appropriated $3 billion to combat bioterrorism, including more than $1 billion to improve state and local public health capabilities and hospital preparedness.

### The Robert Wood Johnson Foundation's Role in Emergency Preparedness

When the anthrax attacks became news in October 2001, the Foundation staff took to the phones, as it had done after September 11th. Nancy Kaufman, for example, called the heads of the National Association of County and City Health Officials and the Association of Public Health Laboratories to ask if they needed help getting information out to the public. They both said yes, and the Foundation provided assistance, similar to that which it had provided in the immediate aftermath of September 11th, to both organizations. Scott Becker, executive director of the Association of Public Health Laboratories, said, "We were deluged. The Foundation's quick response was critical. It not only got us through the immediate crisis but also helped us to develop a long-range communications strategy."

This was a stopgap measure to solve an immediate problem. For the longer term, the Foundation appointed a bioterrorism working group chaired by its two senior vice presidents, Risa Lavizzo-Mourey (now the Foundation's president) and Michael McGinnis, charged with developing a cohesive strategy.[21]

As in the case of September 11th, the Foundation waited to see what the federal government would do. Even as the Foundation grappled to find its niche, however, it made a number of grants that related to the public health system's capacity to deal with bioterrorism.

One cluster of grants helped organizations trying to understand biological terror and to chart a course of action in responding to it. These included awards to conduct public opinion surveys; to hold meetings or disseminate results of meetings on bioterrorism; to add sessions on bioterrorism to previously planned meetings; and to establish a collaborative network of academic and research organizations that would design ways to respond to public health emergencies.

A second cluster of grants went to organizations working on communications and getting information out to the public. The Annenberg School for Communications was awarded a grant to improve journalists' coverage of terrorism; Burness Communications received funding to follow up its work with the Association of State and Territorial Health Officials, the National Association of County and City Health Officials, and the Association of Public Health Laboratories, and raise awareness of the importance of rebuilding the public health infrastructure; the Trust for America's Health received funds to develop an educational campaign to build support for strengthening the public health system.

Additionally, working through both past and new grantees, the Foundation sought to strengthen the ability of practitioners and public health officials to deal with public health emergencies:

- In July 2002, America's Health Together was awarded a half-million-dollar grant to hold workshops and design materials that would strengthen the ability of primary care practitioners to provide mental health services, especially to those affected by terrorism.

- Turning Point, a program that the W. K. Kellogg Foundation and The Robert Wood Johnson Foundation have funded since 1996, has the express purpose of strengthening the public health infrastructure. Building on relationships forged under the program in twenty-three states, state and local officials were able to work together in preparing the comprehensive statewide emergency preparation plans needed to obtain federal bioterrorism funds early in 2002.[22]

- The State Health Leadership Initiative is another Foundation-funded program aimed at strengthening the nation's public health system. Through the National Governors Association, it provides orientation and training for state health department officials. The opportunity for state health officers to meet their counterparts from other states, before the anthrax attacks, made it easier to work across state lines after those acts of bioterrorism.

- The Foundation greatly expanded a small program of the Public Health Informatics Institute originally designed to help states with their information technology needs. After Congress appropriated money, in December 2001, to combat bioterrorism, public health departments and public health laboratories were inundated with people wanting to sell them all sorts of information and communications products. Few had the capacity to make wise choices among the many possibilities of hardware and software. So, in September 2002, the Foundation awarded the Institute $2.8 million (1) to provide health departments with unbiased analyses (a kind of *Consumer Reports*) of the information technology available to respond to bioterrorism and similar public health emergencies; and (2) in combination with the Association of Public Health Laboratories, to collaborate in the development of requirements for upgrading public health laboratories' information systems.

The Foundation continues to make grants to help public health agencies prepare for bioterror emergencies. However, by the middle of 2002, the bioterrorism task force had pretty much dissolved, and its work merged into that of a staff team devoted to improving the health of populations. With a reorganization of the Foundation early in 2003, bioterrorism preparedness had been placed within a staff team whose priority was improving public health leadership and capacity.

## —ɯ— Issues and Reflections

September 11th and the anthrax attacks that followed forced the United States to recognize that a strong public health system is vital to national security, and it forced The Robert Wood Johnson Foundation to rethink how it should respond to emergencies. In earlier days, in the aftermath of a natural disaster, the Foundation simply wrote a check to the American

Red Cross or some other charitable organization to help with the relief effort. The overwhelming public response to September 11th rendered that kind of approach irrelevant and left the Foundation to work, for the most part, on the margins. The anthrax attacks and what they revealed about the weaknesses in the public health infrastructure gave the Foundation an opportunity to craft a cohesive strategy. As senior program officer Susan Hassmiller said, "September 11th and the anthrax attacks forced us to take a systematic approach to disasters rather than responding on an ad hoc basis as we have done in the past." While the Foundation has not yet succeeded in developing a strategic way to deal with emergencies, in its efforts to do so, it has been forced to grapple with a number of important issues, such as those discussed in the following paragraphs.

### Finding an Appropriate Role

The Robert Wood Johnson Foundation has, since its earliest days, funded demonstration programs with the idea of highlighting a good idea, testing its value, and inducing the federal government to replicate it on a national scale. Terrorism, and particularly bioterrorism, turns this on its head. The massive amount of federal aid dwarfs the resources that any single foundation—indeed, all foundations combined—can contribute. In a real sense, the federal government has preempted the field.

In the cases of both the September 11th and the anthrax attacks, the Foundation's response was to proceed cautiously as it searched for a role. It waited to see what others would do and looked to fill the gaps. While caution may be appropriate, it bucks a long tradition, dating back to the establishment of a national emergency medical response system in the 1970s, of the Foundation's taking a leadership role as it collaborated with the federal government on matters of great import to the nation's health. The Robert Wood Johnson Foundation often helped shape the direction a field took and used its relative flexibility to fund activities the government couldn't or wouldn't.[23] In the case of emergency preparation and response, the Foundation did not do this. Nor did it use its stature fully to serve as neutral convener. As the Public Health Informatics Institute's director David Ross noted, "Public health is, to a great extent, a federal enterprise, with funds being allotted on a disease-by-disease basis. September 11$^{th}$ demonstrated that public health had to act as collective enterprise. Bringing people together would have been an appropriate role for the Foundation to play."

Perhaps the lesson from this is that there needs to be a rethinking about the role of a foundation in situations where the scope of an emergency, or a potential emergency, is so great and the infusion of federal government resources (or voluntary contributions) is so enormous that it appears at first glance to marginalize the activities of all others.

### Balancing Long-Term Strategic Objectives and Short-Term Compassionate Responses

While foundations do not want to be, or even appear to be, hard-hearted in helping victims of hurricanes, earthquakes, or terrorist attacks, they also must recognize that money used for immediate compassionate purposes will not be available to further the long-term goals of the foundation. And they must also recognize that Americans respond generously to the immediacy of a disaster, whereas their compassion and generosity are not so easily triggered by long-run systemic social problems. Considering this issue, former Foundation president Steven Schroeder observed, "We need to retain the flexibility to respond to crises, but we must also remain faithful to our core, long-term interests."

This argues for a proportionate response to disasters, especially natural disasters, that shows compassion but does not divert too much money from long-range objectives. Donations in the form of grants to the American Red Cross and other charitable organizations to support relief efforts for victims of natural disasters, for example, are appropriate, although the capricious way (one that depends to a great extent on whether a request has come to the attention of a responsive staff member) they have been given in the past is questionable. Rather than making a grant in the wake of a specific hurricane, flood, or earthquake, it might make sense to consider earmarking an annual contribution to the Red Cross (or other charity) that can be used for disaster relief at the agency's discretion. That way, the Foundation would not have to pick and choose among disasters and the Red Cross (or other organization) would know it can count on a stable source of funds to use in emergencies wherever they occur.

### Weighing Broad and Narrow Approaches to Public Health and Public Health Emergencies

In focusing on the next steps, should attention be given to the broader objective of strengthening the public health system as a whole, the narrower objective of strengthening the system's ability to respond to a biological terror attack, or the medium objective of strengthening the system's capacity to respond to outbreaks of infectious diseases (whether occurring naturally or intentionally)?

Major federal funding to strengthen the public health system's ability to respond to a bioterror incident may have an ancillary benefit— strengthening the system's capacity to identify and address outbreaks of infectious diseases, such as West Nile virus or SARS, not caused by terrorists. It does little to shore up, and is even likely to divert resources from, the public health system's traditional roles, such as protecting mother-child health, combating chronic illnesses, and providing preventive health services to those in need. As the American Public Health Association noted, "It is also important that funding for bioterrorism preparedness does not supplant resources needed for other important public health activities."[24] Yet this is exactly what is happening.[25]

To prevent further deterioration of the system, a focus on public health as a whole, while not neglecting bioterrorism, might be appropriate. Whether The Robert Wood Johnson Foundation chooses to focus narrowly on bioterrorism or more broadly on public health, it is in a position to provide intellectual energy and moral direction, as it has in the past, to a field that is being increasingly recognized as critically important to the nation's well-being.

## Notes

1. Seessel, T. *The Philanthropic Response to 9/11.* (Unpublished). Report prepared for the Ford Foundation, 2002, p. ii.

2. *September 11: Perspectives from the Field of Philanthropy.* The Foundation Center, 2002, p. 110.

3. *Giving in the Aftermath of 9/11.* The Foundation Center, 2002, p. 3.

4. Greene, S. G. "In Disaster's Wake." *Chronicle of Philanthropy,* Sept. 5, 2002, p. 8.

5. Controversy about the use of funds raised by the American Red Cross led to the resignation of its chief executive officer, Bernadine Healy, and to changes in the way it allocates money raised in response to specific emergencies. See Sontag, D. "Who Brought Bernadine Healy Down?" *New York Times,* Dec. 23, 2001.

6. *September 11: Interim Report on the Response of Charities.* Report no. GAO-02–1037. U.S. General Accounting Office, 2002.

7. As of the end of 2002, the fund had settled 142 cases, ranging from $250,000 to more than $3 million. Cukan, A. "2002 Yearend: What's a WTC Life Worth?" United Press International, Dec. 24, 2002. (www.upi.com).

8. Haslanger, K. "Radical Simplification: Disaster Relief Medicaid in New York City." *Health Affairs,* 2003, *22*(1), 252–258.

9. Hensley, S. "Follow the Money." *Wall Street Journal,* Nov. 12, 2002.

10. The program is described in Wielawski, I. M. "The Local Initiative Funding Partners Program." In *To Improve Health and Health Care 2000: The Robert Wood Johnson Foundation Anthology.* San Francisco: Jossey-Bass, 2000.

11. Baker, A. "In Crisis, Its Past Hampered the Office of Emergency Management." *New York Times,* Sept. 9, 2002, p. A13.

12. Worth, R. F. "Uphill Fight for a Downtown Volunteer." *New York Times,* Feb. 11, 2002, p. B1.

13. Preston, R. *The Demon in the Freezer.* New York: Random House, 2002, pp. 1–9.

14. O'Toole, T., Inglesby, T. V., and Henderson, D. A. "Why Understanding Biological Weapons Matters to Medical and Public Health Professionals." In D. A. Henderson, T. V. Inglesby, and T. O'Toole (eds.), *Bioterrorism: Guidelines for Medical and Public Health Management.* Chicago: American Medical Association, 2002, pp. 1–6.

15. This chapter refers to preparation for and responding to biological terrorism. However, the same readiness is needed for other, similar

kinds of attacks: chemical, radiological, or nuclear. In some cases, *bioterrorism* is used as a shorthand for terrorism involving biological, chemical, radiological, and nuclear weapons.

16. Goldberg, J. "The Great Terror." *New Yorker,* Mar. 25, 2002.

17. Miller, J., Engelberg, S., and Broad, W. *Germs: Biological Weapons and America's Secret War.* New York: Simon & Schuster, 2001, p. 175.

18. Institute of Medicine. *The Future of Public Health.* Washington, D.C.: National Academy Press, 1988.

19. Frist, B. *When Every Moment Counts.* Lanham, Md.: Rowman & Littlefield, 2002, pp. 166–167.

20. Lurie, N. "The Public Health Infrastructure: Rebuild or Redesign?" *Health Affairs,* 2002, *21,* 28–30.

21. In 2002, the work of the bioterrorism working group became part of the Foundation's program management team devoted to improving population health.

22. Bekemeier, B., and Dahl, J. "Turning Point Sets the Stage for Bioterrorism Preparedness." *Transformations in Public Health,* Autumn 2002.

23. Editors' Introduction to this volume.

24. *One Year After the Terrorist Attacks: Is Public Health Prepared? A Report Card from the American Public Health Association.* American Public Health Association, 2002.

25. Altman, L., and O'Connor, A. "Health Officials Fear Local Impact of Smallpox Plan." *New York Times,* Jan. 5, 2003.

# -ɯɯ-The Editors

*Stephen L. Isaacs,* J.D., is the president of Health Policy Associates in San Francisco and a principal in the consulting firm of Isaacs/Jellinek. A former professor of public health at Columbia University and founding director of its Development Law and Policy Program, he has written extensively for professional and popular audiences. His book *The Consumer's Legal Guide to Today's Health Care* was reviewed as "the single best guide to the health care system in print today." His articles have been widely syndicated and have appeared in law reviews and health policy journals. He also provides technical assistance internationally on health law, civil society, and social policy. A graduate of Brown University and Columbia Law School, Isaacs served as vice president of International Planned Parenthood's Western Hemisphere Region, practiced health law, and spent four years in Thailand as a program officer for the U.S. Agency for International Development.

*James R. Knickman,* Ph.D., is vice president for research and evaluation at The Robert Wood Johnson Foundation. He oversees a range of grants and national programs supporting research and policy analysis to better understand forces that can improve health status and delivery of health care. In addition, he is in charge of developing formal evaluations of national programs supported by the Foundation. He also has played a leadership role in developing grantmaking strategies in the area of chronic illness during his tenure at the Foundation. During the 1999–2000 academic year, he held a Regents' Lectureship at the University of California, Berkeley. Previously, Knickman was on the faculty of the Robert Wagner Graduate School of Public Service at New York University. At

NYU, he was the founding director of a university-wide research center focused on urban health care. His publications include research on a range of health care topics, with particular emphasis on issues related to financing and delivering long-term care. He has served on numerous health-related advisory committees at the state and local levels and spent a year working at New York City's Office of Management and Budget. Currently, he chairs the board of trustees of Robert Wood Johnson University Hospital. He completed his undergraduate work at Fordham University and received his doctorate in public policy analysis from the University of Pennsylvania.

# –ɯ–The Contributors

*Arlyss Anderson Rothman,* Ph.D., M.H.S., R.N.-C.S., F.N.P., is assistant professor of family health care nursing in the School of Nursing, University of California, San Francisco. She has a doctorate in organizational theory and health services delivery and a master's degree in health services. Anderson Rothman has worked in primary care as a family nurse practitioner and educator for over twenty-five years and has been conducting health services research for five years. Her studies have included nurse practitioner practice in California, the future of medical education in California, interdisciplinary health care teams in ambulatory care, residents' attitudes toward fellowship training, the future of primary care in the United States, and the need for nurse management training programs. Anderson Rothman maintains a private practice as a family nurse practitioner in Berkeley, California.

*Paul Brodeur* was a staff writer at the *New Yorker* for nearly forty years. During that time, he alerted the nation to the public health hazard posed by asbestos, to depletion of the ozone layer by chlorofluorocarbons, and to the harmful effects of microwave radiation and power-frequency electromagnetic fields. His work has been acknowledged with a National Magazine Award and the Journalism Award of the American Association for the Advancement of Science. The United Nations Environment Program has named him to its Global 500 Roll of Honour for outstanding environmental achievements.

*Ethan Bronner* is the assistant editorial page editor of the *New York Times.* From 1999 through 2001 he was the paper's education editor. He came to the *New York Times* in 1997 as a national correspondent and reported on trends in higher education and grades K–12. From 1985 until 1997 he was with the *Boston Globe,* where he served as Middle East correspondent, based in Jerusalem, and a Supreme Court and legal affairs correspondent in Washington, D.C. He began his journalistic career at Reuters in 1980 and reported from London, Madrid, and Brussels. Bronner is the author of *Battle for Justice: How the Bork Nomination Shook America,* which was chosen by the New York Public Library as one of the twenty-five best books of 1989. He received a B.A. in letters from Wesleyan University and an M.S. from Columbia University's School of Journalism.

*Digby Diehl* is a writer, literary collaborator, and television, print, and Internet journalist. Recently honored with the Jack Smith Award from the Friends of the Pasadena Public Library, his book credits include *Angel on My Shoulder,* the autobiography of singer Natalie Cole; *The Million Dollar Mermaid,* the autobiography of MGM star Esther Williams; *Tales from the Crypt,* the history of the popular comic book, movie, and television series; and *A Spy for All Seasons,* the autobiography of former CIA officer Duane Clarridge. For eleven years, Diehl was the literary correspondent for ABC-TV's *Good Morning America* and was recently the book editor for the *Home Page* show on MSNBC. He continues to appear regularly on the morning news on KTLA. Previously the entertainment editor for KCBS television in Los Angeles, he was a writer for the Emmys and for the soap opera *Santa Barbara,* book editor of the *Los Angeles Herald Examiner,* editor in chief of art book publisher Harry N. Abrams, and the founding book editor of the *Los Angeles Times Book Review.* Diehl holds an M.A. in theatre from UCLA and a B.A. in American studies from Rutgers University, where he was a Henry Rutgers Scholar. He is presently collaborating with Coretta Scott King on her memoirs.

*Richard S. Frank* is a freelance writer and editor and is currently an adjunct professor at Boston University's Washington Journalism Center. From 1976 to 1997 he was the editor of *National Journal,* the Washington-based weekly on national politics and federal policy. During his tenure, the magazine won two National Magazine Awards, and its reporters won numerous national awards for public affairs reporting. His earlier journalistic experience included stints as a local government reporter for the *Bergen Record* in New Jersey, as a statehouse and city hall reporter for the *Baltimore Evening Sun*, as state legislative correspondent and public transportation reporter, and later as a Washington correspondent, for the *Philadelphia Bulletin*, and as international economics and trade reporter, associate editor, and managing editor at *National Journal.* He interrupted his journalistic career for almost two years to serve as chief administrative assistant to the mayor of Baltimore. He has a bachelor's degree from Syracuse University in international relations and journalism and a master's degree from the University of Chicago in political science, and he was an Advanced International Reporting Fellow at Columbia University.

*Paul Jellinek,* Ph.D., is a principal at Isaacs/Jellinek and senior fellow at Health Policy Associates. He served on the staff of The Robert Wood Johnson Foundation from 1983 to 2002, the last eleven years as a vice president for programs. At the Foundation, he was involved in developing and managing programs to improve access to health care, reduce the harm from substance abuse, and improve the organization and delivery of chronic care services. Jellinek has had a particular interest in developing programs to strengthen community capacity, including Fighting Back and Join Together. A former fellow at the Bush Institute for Child and Family Policy in North Carolina, his articles have appeared in the *New England Journal of Medicine, Health Affairs,* and *Issues in Science and Technology.* Jellinek received a Ph.D. in health policy and administration with a concentration in health economics, as well as a master's degree in health administration, from the School of Public Health at the University of North Carolina at Chapel Hill. He is a graduate of the University of Pennsylvania and the University of South Florida.

*Risa Lavizzo-Mourey,* M.D., MBA, joined the staff of The Robert Wood Johnson Foundation in April 2001 as the senior vice president and director of the health care group. In January 2003, she became the Foundation's fourth president and chief executive officer. Prior to coming to the Foundation, Lavizzo-Mourey was the Sylvan Eisman Professor of Medicine and Health Care Systems at the University of Pennsylvania. Lavizzo-Mourey served as the deputy administrator of the Agency for Health Care Policy and Research (now the Agency for Health Care Research and Quality). While in government service, she worked on the White House health care policy team, including the White House Task Force on Health Care Reform, where she co-chaired the working group on quality of care. Lavizzo-Mourey has served on numerous federal advisory committees and is a member of the Institute of Medicine of the National Academy of Sciences and a Master of the American College of Physicians–American Society of Internal Medicine. She earned her medical degree at Harvard Medical School and a MBA degree at the University of Pennsylvania's Wharton School. After completing a residency in internal medicine at Brigham and Women's Hospital in Boston, Lavizzo-Mourey was a Robert Wood Johnson Clinical Scholar at the University of Pennsylvania, where she also received her geriatrics training.

*Laura C. Leviton,* Ph.D., is a senior program officer at The Robert Wood Johnson Foundation. Before joining the Foundation, she was a professor of public health at the University of Alabama at Birmingham and before that, on the faculty of the University of Pittsburgh School of Public Health. Leviton is a leading writer on evaluation methods and practice, in particular for disease prevention. She was president of the American Evaluation Association in 2000, coauthored a leading evaluation text, and serves on several editorial boards for evaluation journals. She received the 1993 award from the American Psychological Association for Distinguished Contributions to Psychology in the Public Interest for her work in HIV prevention and health promotion in the workplace. She served on an Institute of Medicine committee to evaluate preparedness for terrorist attacks, and was a member of the CDC's National Advisory Committee on HIV and STD Prevention.

*Jane Isaacs Lowe,* Ph.D., is a senior program officer at The Robert Wood Johnson Foundation and serves as the team leader for the vulnerable populations portfolio, a program staff group focused on improving social health outcomes for low-income children, families, and older adults. At the Foundation, she is also responsible for the development of minority health professions training programs and a matching grants program with local funding partners. She is a current fellow at the New York Academy of Medicine and a member of the board of Grantmakers in Aging. Lowe came to the Foundation from the University of Pennsylvania School of Social Work, where she served as a member of the faculty from 1989 to 1998. She was the recipient of the Outstanding Teaching Award in 1992 and 1997. From 1976 to 1989 she worked at the Mt. Sinai Medical Center (New York City), where she served as a faculty member in the medical school's Department of Community Medicine and as a hospital social work administrator. Lowe has extensive experience in chronic illness, community-based health, and program planning. She earned her bachelor's degree in sociology and education from Cedar Crest College, her master's degree in social work from Columbia University, and her doctorate in social welfare policy and planning from Rutgers University.

*Carolyn Newbergh* is a Northern California writer who has covered health care trends and policy issues for more than twenty years. Her freelance work has appeared in numerous print and on-line publications. As a reporter for the *Oakland Tribune,* she wrote articles on health care delivery for the poor as well as emergency room violence, AIDS, and the impact of crack cocaine on the children of addicts. She was also an investigative reporter for the *Tribune,* winning prestigious honors for a series on how consultants intentionally cover up earthquake hazards in California.

*Constance M. Pechura,* Ph.D., is a senior program officer at The Robert Wood Johnson Foundation, responsible for the Foundation's Minority Medical Faculty Development Program, Community Health Leadership Program, Health Policy Fellowships Program, and Depression in Primary Care Program. She came to the Foundation from the Institute of Medicine/National Academies of Science, where she directed a number of studies in health sciences policy, neuroscience and behavioral health, and veterans' health, as a senior staff officer from 1988 to 1993. Pechura also served as deputy director (from 1993 to 1995) and director (from 1995 to 1998) of the institute's Board on Neuroscience and Behavioral Health. In addition, she taught health policy in the Stanford in Washington Program from 1993 to 1998, and anatomy and neuroscience courses at George

Washington University Medical School and the F. Edward Hebert School of Medicine at the Uniformed Services University of the Health Sciences (USUHS). Pechura earned a B.S. in psychology at Virginia Common-wealth University and a Ph.D. in anatomy, with a specialization in neuro-science, from USUHS. Her awards include a National Science Foundation Graduate Fellowship, an Outstanding Teaching award from the USUHS Medical School Class of 1988, and the National Research Council's Spe-cial Achievement Award in 1993.

*Lewis G. Sandy,* M.D., is executive vice president, Clinical Strategies and Policy, UnitedHealthcare. At UnitedHealthcare, a diversified health and well-being company, he leads efforts to promote efficient and effective health care, provide tools and information to doctors and patients to pro-mote health, and foster the growth of evidence-based medicine. Until 2003, Sandy was executive vice president of The Robert Wood Johnson Foundation, where he was responsible for the Foundation's program de-velopment and management, strategic planning, and administrative operations. Between 1991 and 1996, Sandy was a vice president of the Foundation and was active in the Foundation's workforce initiatives, its efforts to track the changing health care system, its programs to improve services for chronically ill people, and its programs to improve managed care. An internist and former health center medical director at the Har-vard Community Health Plan in Boston, Massachusetts, Sandy received his B.S. and M.D. from the University of Michigan and an M.B.A. from Stanford University. A former Robert Wood Johnson Foundation Clinical Scholar and Clinical Fellow in Medicine at the University of California, San Francisco, Sandy served his internship and residency at the Beth Is-rael Hospital in Boston. He is an associate clinical professor of medicine at the University of Medicine and Dentistry of New Jersey/Robert Wood Johnson Medical School.

*Renie Schapiro* has an extensive background in health writing and policy. She was editor of *The New Physician* magazine and the *Kennedy Institute of Ethics Journal.* She is coeditor of three books, the most recent of which is *Transplanting Human Tissue: Ethics, Policy and Practise* (2003). She was also speechwriter and policy adviser to FDA commissioner David Kessler and a research associate with the President's Commission on Ethical Problems in Medicine and Biomedical Research. She has taught health policy and bioethics at Yale University and the University of Wisconsin–Madison. She was a special communications officer at The Robert Wood Johnson Foundation and over the past several years has been a consultant to the Foundation, working closely with presidents Steven Schroeder and Risa Lavizzo-Mourey on speeches and papers on health policy and philanthropy. She has an M.P.H from Yale University and a B.A. from the University of Minnesota.

*Jonathan Showstack,* Ph.D., M.P.H., is professor of medicine and health policy in the Institute for Health Policy Studies and Department of Medicine, School of Medicine, University of California, San Francisco. He is also associate director of the Institute. Showstack has conducted numerous studies of the costs, effectiveness, and outcomes of medical care and medical education. He has over two decades of experience in the assessment of health care technologies, including studies of kidney and liver transplantation, coronary artery bypass graft surgery, hepatic surgery, neonatal intensive care, and emergency care. He received his doctorate in sociology from the University of California, San Francisco, and his master of public health degree in health administration and planning from the University of California, Berkeley.

*Irene M. Wielawski* is a health care journalist with twenty years' experience on daily newspapers, including the *Providence Journal-Bulletin* and the *Los Angeles Times,* where she was a member of the investigations team. She has written extensively on problems of access to care among the poor and uninsured, and other socioeconomic issues in American medicine. From 1994 through 2000 Wielawski—with a research grant from The Robert Wood Johnson Foundation—tracked the experiences of the medically uninsured in twenty-five states following the demise of President Clinton's health reform plan. Other projects in health care journalism since then have included helping to develop a pediatric medicine program for public television, and freelance assignments for the *New York Times* and the *Los Angeles*

*Times.* Wielawski has been a finalist for the Pulitzer Prize for medical reporting, among other solo honors. She is a founder of the Association of Health Care Journalists and a graduate of Vassar College.

# –ɯ–Index

## A

AAMC (Association of American Medical Colleges): early efforts to increase minority enrollment by, 127–128; Health Professionals for Diversity coalition by, 142–143; Project 3000 by 2000 launched by, 134–135; "underrepresented minorities" definition by, 138, 139, 142

AAMC task force report (1978), 132

AcademyHealth (Washington, D.C.), 76–77

Advocacy/Policy Program, 212

Affirmative action programs, 129–130, 138

Affordable health care: CPAHC (Community Programs for Affordable Health Care) promoting, 67–72; Faculty Fellowships in Health Care Finance programs and, 62, 75–76; importance/frustration of providing, 78–80; Physician-Directed Program to provide, 72–74; prepaid managed health care for, 74–75; risk adjustment concept and, 77–78; skepticism regarding cooperative community approach to, 69–70. *See also* Health care costs

AFL–CLO, 69

African Americans: decreased number applying to medical school, 131; study on child burn injury rates for, 183. *See also* Minority students

A.G. Rhodes Nursing Home (Wesley Woods), 85

Agency for Health Care Policy and Research (now Agency for Healthcare Research and Quality), 112–113

Aiken, L., 86–87, 88, 90

Alcohol abuse: prevalence over illegal drug use by, 20; problems with lumping together illegal drug and, 28; programs to prevent *in utero* exposure to, 208–211; Worcester public feeling about, 20. *See also* Substance abuse

Alcohol and Drug Affected Mothers and Infants (California, 1990), 209

Alfred P. Murrah Federal Building (Oklahoma City), 227

Alfred P. Sloan Foundation, 127

Allegheny General Hospital (Pittsburgh), 183–184

Allen, L. S., 234

Altman, D., 67, 68, 69, 75

Altman, S., 150, 151

American Academy of Pediatrics, 189, 232

American Hospital Association, 69

American Medical Association, 69

American Red Cross, 226–227, 229, 230, 235, 236, 243–244, 245, 246

American Red Cross's Liberty Disaster Fund, 230

America's Health Together, 242

AmeriCorps, 210

Amherst, Sir J., 239

Andrew W. Mellon Foundation, 230

Annenberg School of Communications, 242

*Annual Report* (1996), 64

Anthrax attacks (2001), 223, 224, 238–240, 244

Anti-affirmative action backlash, 138

Art Science Research Laboratory, Inc., 233, 234, 235, 236, 237

ASPIRA, 227

Association of Public Health Laboratories, 241, 242, 243

Association of State and Territorial Health Officials, 242

**259**